T0358667

Curbside Consultation in Pediatric GI

in Pediatric GI

49 Clinical Questions

CURBSIDE CONSULTATION IN PEDIATRICS
SERIES

SERIES EDITOR, LISA B. ZAOUTIS, MD

Curbside Consultation
in Pediatric GI

49 Clinical Questions

Edited By

Joel R. Rosh, MD
Director of Pediatric Gastroenterology
Goryeb Children's Hospital/Atlantic Health
Associate Professor of Pediatrics
New Jersey Medical School
Morristown, New Jersey

Athos Bousvaros, MD, MPH
Associate Professor of Pediatrics
Harvard Medical School
Associate Director
Inflammatory Bowel Disease Program
Children's Hospital of Boston
Boston, Massachusetts

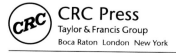

CRC Press
Taylor & Francis Group
Boca Raton London New York

CRC Press is an imprint of the
Taylor & Francis Group, an **informa** business

First published 2013 by SLACK Incorporated

Published 2024 by CRC Press
2385 NW Executive Center Drive, Suite 320, Boca Raton FL 33431

and by CRC Press
4 Park Square, Milton Park, Abingdon, Oxon, OX14 4RN

CRC Press is an imprint of Taylor & Francis Group, LLC

© 2013 Taylor & Francis Group, LLC

This book contains information obtained from authentic and highly regarded sources. While all reasonable efforts have been made to publish reliable data and information, neither the author[s] nor the publisher can accept any legal responsibility or liability for any errors or omissions that may be made. The publishers wish to make clear that any views or opinions expressed in this book by individual editors, authors or contributors are personal to them and do not necessarily reflect the views/opinions of the publishers. The information or guidance contained in this book is intended for use by medical, scientific or health-care professionals and is provided strictly as a supplement to the medical or other professional's own judgement, their knowledge of the patient's medical history, relevant manufacturer's instructions and the appropriate best practice guidelines. Because of the rapid advances in medical science, any information or advice on dosages, procedures or diagnoses should be independently verified. The reader is strongly urged to consult the relevant national drug formulary and the drug companies' and device or material manufacturers' printed instructions, and their websites, before administering or utilizing any of the drugs, devices or materials mentioned in this book. This book does not indicate whether a particular treatment is appropriate or suitable for a particular individual. Ultimately it is the sole responsibility of the medical professional to make his or her own professional judgements, so as to advise and treat patients appropriately. The authors and publishers have also attempted to trace the copyright holders of all material reproduced in this publication and apologize to copyright holders if permission to publish in this form has not been obtained. If any copyright material has not been acknowledged please write and let us know so we may rectify in any future reprint.

Except as permitted under U.S. Copyright Law, no part of this book may be reprinted, reproduced, transmitted, or utilized in any form by any electronic, mechanical, or other means, now known or hereafter invented, including photocopying, microfilming, and recording, or in any information storage or retrieval system, without written permission from the publishers.

For permission to photocopy or use material electronically from this work, access www.copyright.com or contact the Copyright Clearance Center, Inc. (CCC), 222 Rosewood Drive, Danvers, MA 01923, 978-750-8400. For works that are not available on CCC please contact mpkbookspermissions@tandf.co.uk

Trademark notice: Product or corporate names may be trademarks or registered trademarks and are used only for identification and explanation without intent to infringe.

Library of Congress Cataloging-in-Publication Data

Curbside consultation in pediatric GI : 49 clinical questions / [edited by] Joel R. Rosh, Athos Bousvaros.
    p. ; cm. -- (Curbside consultation series)
  Includes bibliographical references and index.
  ISBN 978-1-61711-014-6 (alk. paper)
  I. Rosh, Joel R. II. Bousvaros, Athos. III. Series: Curbside consultation in pediatrics series.
  [DNLM: 1. Gastrointestinal Diseases--diagnosis. 2. Child. 3. Gastrointestinal Diseases--therapy. 4. Infant. 5. Pediatrics--methods. WS 310]

  618.92'330076--dc23
                        2012043727

  ISBN: 9781617110146 (pbk)
  ISBN: 9781003523635 (ebk)

DOI: 10.1201/9781003523635

Dedication

To my parents for giving me the foundation; to Susan for her wise guidance and abundant love; to my children, Dani, Jeremy, and Alex, for making everything worthwhile; and to my patients and their families for teaching me about courage and caring.

—Joel R. Rosh, MD

I would like to dedicate this book to my wife Meg, son George, parents George and Olga, and to Dr. Alan Leichtner.

—Athos Bousvaros, MD, MPH

Contents

Acknowledgments

We would like to thank Dr. Frank Farraye, who gave us the opportunity to edit this book, and to the many wonderful contributors who worked so hard to make this book a reality. Dr. Bousvaros would also like to acknowledge the Rasmussen, Macinnes, Ward, Wolfman, Clark, and Poreda families who have supported his academic work. Dr. Rosh would like to the thank the Goryeb and Rudd families for their continued generosity and support.

About the Editors

Joel R. Rosh, MD graduated from Brown University and received his medical degree from the Albert Einstein College of Medicine in New York. His postdoctoral training included a pediatric residency at the Children's Hospital of New York—Columbia Presbyterian Medical Center and a Clinical Fellowship in Pediatric Gastroenterology at the Mount Sinai Hospital in New York. He has been on the faculty of the University of Medicine and Dentistry of New Jersey, as well as the medical schools of Mount Sinai and New York's Columbia Presbyterian Hospital. Dr. Rosh is a Fellow of the American Academy of Pediatrics (FAAP), the American College of Gastroenterology (FACG), and the American Gastroenterological Association (AGAF). He has served as a National Counselor for the North American Society of Pediatric Gastroenterology, Hepatology, and Nutrition (NASPGHAN), and as the National Chairman of the Pediatric Education Committee for the Crohn's and Colitis Foundation of America (CCFA).

Athos Bousvaros, MD, MPH obtained his BA from Williams College, MD from Duke University School of Medicine, and completed a Master's of Public Health at the Harvard University School of Public Health. After completing his pediatric residency at Duke, he trained in the Combined Program in pediatric gastroenterology and nutrition at Boston Children's Hospital and Massachusetts General Hospital. He is currently the Associate Director of the Inflammatory Bowel Disease Program at Boston Children's Hospital, and an Associate Professor of Pediatrics at Harvard Medical School. Dr. Bousvaros is currently the President of the North American Society of Pediatric Gastroenterology and Nutrition (NASPGHAN). Dr. Bousvaros spends what little spare time he has with his family and his comic book collection. He would like to thank his patients, who are also his greatest teachers.

Contributing Authors

Lindsey Albenberg, DO (Question 39)
Fellow
Divison of Gastrenterology, Hepatology,
  and Nutrition
The Children's Hospital of Philadelphia
Philadelphia, Pennsylvania

Lusine Ambartsumyan, MD (Question 13)
Fellow in Pediatric Gastroenterology and
  Nutrition
Boston Children's Hospital Harvard
Medical School
Boston, Massachussetts

Robert N. Baldassano, MD (Question 39)
Colman Family Chair in Pediatric
  Inflammatory Bowel Disease
Professor, University of Pennsylvania
  School of Medicine
Director, Center for Pediatric
  Inflammatory Bowel Disease
The Children's Hospital of Philadelphia
Phildelphia, Pennsylvania

William F. Balistreri, MD (Question 21)
Medical Director, Emeritus, Pediatric
  Liver Care Center
Division of Pediatric Gastroenterology,
  Hepatology, and Nutrition
Cincinnati Children's Hospital
Professor of Pediatrics, University of
  Cincinnati College of Medicine
Cincinnati, Ohio

Warren P. Bishop, MD (Question 14)
Director, Division of Gastroenterology
University of Iowa Children's Hospital
Professor of Pediatrics
Carver College of Medicine
University of Iowa
Iowa City, Iowa

Samra S. Blanchard, MD (Question 34)
Director of Pediatric Gastroenterology
University Maryland Medical Center
Associate Professor of Pediatrics,
University of Maryland School of
  Medicine
Baltimore, Maryland

Silvana Bonilla, MD (Questions 4, 35)
Assistant Professor of Pediatrics
The Floating Hospital for Children at Tufts
  Medical Center
Boston, Massachusetts

Timothy M. Buie, MD (Question 49)
Assisatant Professor of Pediatrics, Harvard
  Medical School
Associate Pediatrician, Massachusetts
  General Hospital for Children
Boston, Massachusetts

Ashley Casserino, MD (Question 20)
Pediatric Resident
Connecticut Children's Medical Center
University of Connecticut Health Center
Hartford, Connecticut

Kathy D. Chen, MD (Question 26)
Assistant Professor of Pediatrics
Drexel University College of Medicine
St. Christopher's Hospital for Children
Philadelphia, Pennsylvania

Peter Church, MD (Question 42)
Pediatric IBD Fellow
Division of Gastroenterology, Hepatology,
  and Nutrition
Department of Pediatrics
SickKids Hospital
University of Toronto
Toronto, Ontario

Wallace Crandall, MD (Question 45)
Director, The Center for Pediatric and
    Adolescent Inflammatory Bowel
    Disease
Associate Medical Director for Quality
Nationwide Children's Hospital
Professor of Clinical Pediatrics
The Ohio State University College of
    Medicine
Columbus, Ohio

*Steven J. Czinn, MD, FAAP, FACG, AGAF
    (Question 34)*
Professor and Chair
Department of Pediatrics, University of
    Maryland School of Medicine
Physician-in-Chief, University of Maryland
    Children's Hospital
Baltimore, Maryland

Marla Dubinsky, MD (Question 44)
Director, Pediatric Inflammatory Bowel
    Disease Program
Associate Professor of Pediatrics
Cedars-Sinai Medical Center
Los Angeles, California

Jaime Echartea, MD (Question 21)
Assistant Professor, Department of
    Pediatrics
Division of Gastroenterology, Hepatology,
    and Nutrition
UT Health Science Center
San Antonio, Texas

Steven H. Erdman, MD (Question 47)
Professor of Clinical Pediatrics
Nationwide Children's Hospital
The Ohio State University College of
    Medicine
Columbus, Ohio

Douglas G. Field, MD (Question 6)
Professor of Pediatrics
Director of Pediatric Gastroenterology,
    Hepatology, and Nutrition
Penn State Hershey Children's Hospital
Hershey, Pennsylvania

Thomas Flass, MD, MS (Question 29)
Pediatric Gastroenterology
Fortin Pediatric Specialty Clinic
St. Vincent Healthcare
Billings, Montana

Alejandro F. Flores, MD (Question 4)
Director of Pediatric Gastroenterology
The Floating Hospital for Children at
    Tufts Medical Center
Professor of Pediatrics
Boston, Massachusetts

Glenn T. Furuta, MD (Question 32)
Professor of Pediatrics
Director Gastrointestinal Eosinophilic
    Diseases Program
Digestive Health Institute
Section of Gastroenterology, Hepatology,
    and Nutrition
Children's Hospital Colorado
Gastrointestinal Eosinophilic Diseases
    Program
National Jewish Health
University of Colorado School of Medicine
Aurora, Colorado

*Benjamin D. Gold, MD, FAAP, FACG
    (Question 33)*
Children's Center for Digestive Healthcare
Pediatric Gastroenterology, Hepatology,
    and Nutrition
Atlanta, Georgia

Tanja Gonska, MD (Question 24)
Assistant Professor
Division of Gastroenterology, Hepatology,
    and Nutrition
University of Toronto
Associate Scientist, Research Institute
The Hospital for Sick Children
Ontario, Canada

Nidhi P. Goyal, MD, MPH (Question 17)
Pediatric Gastroenterology Fellow
Division of Pediatric Gastroenterology,
    Hepatology, and Nutrition
Rady Children's Hospital
University of California
San Diego, California

Anne M. Griffiths, MD, FRCPC
    (Question 42)
Head, Division of Gastroenterology,
    Hepatology, and Nutrition
Northbridge Chair in Inflammatory Bowel
    Disease
SickKids Hospital
Professor of Pediatrics
University of Toronto
Toronto, Ontario

Stefano Guandalini, MD (Question 38)
Professor, Pediatrics
Chief, Section of Gastroenterology
Founder and Medical Director, Celica
    Disease Center
University of Chicago Comer Children's
    Hospital
Chicago, Illinois

Sandeep Gupta, MD, AGAF, FACG, FASGE,
    FAAP (Question 3)
Professor of Clinical Pediatrics and
    Internal Medicine
Pediatric Gastroenterology, Hepatology,
    and Nutrition
Riley Hospital for Children at Indiana
    University Health
Indianapolis, Indiana

Melvin B. Heyman, MD, MPH (Question 43)
Anita Ow Wing Endowed Chair
Professor of Pediatrics
Director, UCSF Pediatric Inflammatory
    Bowel Disease Program
Chief, Division of Pediatric
    Gastroenterology, Hepatology and
    Nutrition
UCSF Benioff Children's Hospital
University of California
San Francisco, California

Ivor D. Hill, MB, ChB, MD (Question 28)
Professor of Pediatrics and Internal
    Medicine
Chief, Section of Pediatric
    Gastroenterology, Hepatology, and
    Nutrition
Wake Forest University School of Medicine
Winston-Salem, North Carolina

Edward J. Hoffenberg, MD (Question 29)
Professor, Pediatrics
Director, Center for Pediatric
Children's Hospital of Colorado
    Inflammatory Bowel Diseases
University of Colorado Denver School of
    Medicine
Aurora, Colorado

Jeannie Huang, MD, MPH (Question 16)
Associate Professor, Division of Pediatric
    Gastroenterology
Fellowship Director, Program in Pediatric
    Gastroenterology, Hepatology, and
    Nutrition
Rady Children's Hospital/UC San Diego
San Diego, California

Sohail Z. Husain, MD (Question 26)
Associate Professor of Pediatrics
Children's Hospital of Pittsburgh of UPMC
    and the University of Pittsburgh
Pittsburgh, Pennsylvania

Jeffrey S. Hyams, MD (Question 41)
Director of the Division of Digestive
    Diseases, Hepatology, and Nutrition
Connecticut Children's Medical Center
Professor of Pediatrics, University of
    Connecticut School of Medicine
Hartford, Connecticut

Paul E. Hyman, MD (Question 1)
Chief, Pediatric Gastroenterology
Children's Hospital
Professor of Pediatrics
Louisiana State University
New Orleans, Louisiana

Maureen M. Jonas, MD (Question 9)
Director, Center for Childhood Liver
    Disease
Boston Children's Hospital
Professor of Pediatrics, Harvard Medical
    School
Boston, Massachusetts

Subra Kugathasan, MD (Question 40)
Marcus Professor of Pediatric
    Gastroenterology
Professor of Pediatrics and Human
    Genetics
Emory University School of Medicine and
    Children's Healthcare of Atlanta
Atlanta, Georgia

Anayansi Lasso-Pirot, MD (Question 34)
Assistant Professor and Interim Division
    Head
Department of Pediatrics, Division of
    Allergy/Pulmonology
University of Maryland School of
    Medicine
Baltimore, Maryland

Joel E. Lavine, MD, PhD (Question 22)
Professor of Pediatrics
Chief, Pediatric Gastroenterology,
    Hepatology, and Nutrition
Columbia University Medical Center
New York, New York

Dale Y. Lee, MD (Question 48)
Fellow, Division of Pediatric
    Gastroenterology, Hepatology, and
    Nutrition
The Children's Hospital of Philadelphia
Philadelphia, Pennsylvania

Ian Leibowitz, MD (Question 2)
Director of Pediatric Gastroenterology
Director of Pediatric Digestive Disease
    Center
Inova Fairfax Hospital for Children
Fairfax, Virginia

Alan M. Leichtner, MD (Question 30)
Division of Gastroenterology and
    Nutrition
Boston Children's Hospital Harvard
    Medical School
Boston, Massachusetts

Neil S. LeLeiko, MD, PhD (Question 46)
Director, Division of Pediatric
    Gastroenterology, Nutrition, and Liver
    Diseases
Hasbro Children's Hospital/The Rhode
    Island Hospital
Professor, Department of Pediatrics
Alpert School of Medicine at Brown
    University
Providence, Rhode Island

Henry Lin, MD (Question 7)
Division of Pediatric Gastroenterology,
    Hepatology, and Nutrition
The Children's Hospital of Philadelphia
Philadelphia, Pennsylvania

Douglas Lindblad, MD (Question 27)
Children's Hospital of Pittsburgh of
    University of Pittsburgh Medical Center
Assistant Professor of Pediatrics
University of Pittsburgh
Pittsburgh, Pennsylvania

Debra Lobato, PhD (Question 46)
Director, Division of Child Psychology
Department of Psychiatry
Warren Alpert School of Medicine at
  Brown University
Bradley Hasbro Children's Research
  Center
Rhode Island Hospital/Hasbro Children's
  Hospital
Providence, Rhode Island

Vera Loening-Baucke, MD (Question 15)
Professor Emeritus of Pediatrics
University of Iowa
Iowa City, Iowa

Mark E. Lowe, MD, PhD (Question 27)
Director of Gastroenterology, Hepatology,
  and Nutrition
Children's Hospital of Pittsburgh of
  University of Pittsburgh Medical Center
Professor and Vice-Chairman of Pediatrics
University of Pittsburgh
Pittsburgh, Pennsylvania

Laura Mackner, PhD (Question 45)
Investigator, Center for Biobehavioral
  Health
Psychologist, Divison of Pediatric
  Psychology
Nationwide Children's Hospital
Columbus, Ohio

Petar Mamula, MD (Question 48)
Division of Gastroenterology, Hepatology,
  and Nutrition
The Children's Hospital of Philadelphia
Philadelphia, Pennsylvania

Ali A. Mencin, MD (Question 22)
Assistant Professor of Pediatrics
Division of Pediatric Gastroenterology,
  Hepatology, and Nutrition
Columbia University Medical Center
New York, New York

*Sonia K. Michail, MD, CPE, FAAP, AGAF
  (Question 19)*
Associate Professor of Clinical Pediatrics
The University of Southern California
Los Angeles, California

Jeremy P. Middleton, MD (Question 40)
Emory University/Children's Healthcare
  of Atlanta
Fellow, Pediatric Gastroenterology,
  Hepatology, and Nutrition
Atlanta, Georgia

Douglas Mogul, MD, MPH (Question 8)
Fellow, Pediatric Gastroenterology
Johns Hopkins University
Baltimore, Maryland

Michael R. Narkewicz, MD (Question 23)
Professor, Pediatrics
Hewit Andrews Chair, Pediatric Liver
  Diseases
Pediatric Services Associate Clinical
  Director/Associate Dean for Pediatric
  Clinical Affairs
Director, Fellowship Program
Medical Director, Pediatric Liver Center
  and Liver Transplantation
Children's Hospital of Colorado
Aurora, Colorado

Catherine D. Newland, MD (Question 38)
Pediatric Gastroenterology Fellow
University of Chicago, Comer Children's
  Hospital
Chicago, Illinois

Samuel Nurko, MD, MPH (Question 13)
Director Center for Motility and
  Functional Gastrointestinal Disorders
Boston Children's Hospital Associate
Professor of Pediatrics
Harvard Medical School
Boston, Massachusetts

Adam Paul, DO (Question 34)
Fellow, Pediatric Gastroenterology
University of Maryland Children's
   Hospital
Baltimore, Maryland

Emily R. Perito, MD, MAS (Question 43)
Division of Pediatric Gastroenterology,
   Hepatology, and Nutrition
Benioff Children's Hospital
University of California
San Francisco, California

David A. Piccoli, MD (Question 7)
Division of Pediatric Gastroenterology,
   Hepatology, and Nutrition
The Children's Hospital of Philadelphia
Philadelphia, Pennsylvania

Audra S. Rouster, MD (Question 1)
Pediatric Gastroenterology Fellow
Louisiana State University
New Orleans, Louisiana

Colin Rudolph, MD, PhD (Question 5)
Vice-President for Global Medical Affairs
   and Chief Medical Officer
Mead Johnson Nutrition
Evansville, Indiana

Miguel Saps, MD (Question 35)
Director of Functional Bowel and Motility
   Disorders
Lurie Children's Hospital of Chicago
Associate Professor of Pediatrics
Northwestern University, Feinberg School
   of Medicine
Chicago, Illinois

Shauna Schroeder, MD (Question 32)
Faculty in Pediatric Gastroenterology,
   Hepatology, and Nutrition,
Phoenix Children's Hospital
Phoenix, Arizona

Kathleen B. Schwarz, MD (Question 8)
Director, Pediatric Liver Center
Professor of Pediatrics
President, NASPGHAN
Division of Pediatric Gastroenterology,
   Hepatology, and Nutrition
Johns Hopkins University School of
   Medicine
Baltimore, Maryland

Jeffrey B. Schwimmer, MD (Question 17)
Associate Professor, Pediatrics
Division of Gastroenterology, Hepatology,
   and Nutrition
Department of Pediatrics, University of
   California, San Diego
Director, Weight and Wellness
Director, Fatty Liver Clinic
Rady Children's Hospital
San Diego, California

Leigha Senter, MS, CGC
   (Question 47)
Certified Genetic Counselor
Assistant Professor, Internal Medicine
The Ohio State University Medical Center
Ohio State's Comprehensive Cancer
   Center—James Center Hospital and
   Solove Research Institute
Columbus, Ohio

Scott H. Sicherer, MD (Question 31)
Professor, Pediatrics
Jaffe Food Allergy Institute
Mount Sinai School of Medicine
New York, New York

Natalie Sikka, MD (Question 2)
Pediatric Gastroenterologist
Pediatric Digestive Disease Center
Inova Fairfax Hospital for Children
Fairfax, Virginia

Edwin F. Simpser, MD (Question 10)
Chief Medical Officer
St. Mary's Healthcare System for Children
Assistant Professor of Pediatrics
Hofstra North Shore-LIJ School of
    Medicine
Bayside, New York

Frank R. Sinatra, MD (Question 18)
Professor of Pediatrics
Assistant Dean for Faculty Development
Keck School of Medicine
University of Southern California
Los Angeles, California

Namita Singh, MD (Question 44)
Fellow, Pediatric Gastroenterology
Seattle Children's Hospital/University of
    Washington
Seattle, Washington

Judith M. Sondheimer, MD (Question 12)
Professor of Pediatrics
Chief Pediatric Gastroenterology
Georgetown University and Medstar
Georgetown University Hospital
Washington, DC

Janis M. Stoll, MD (Question 9)
Advanced Fellow, Hepatology
Division of Pediatric Gastroenterology,
    Hepatology, and Nutrition
Children's Hospital of Boston
Boston, Massachussetts

Alexander Swidsinski, MD (Question 15)
Director of the Laboratory for Molecular
    Genetics, Polymicrobial Infections, and
    Bacterial Biofilms
Department of Medicine, Section of
    Gastroenterology, Hepatology and
    Endocrinology
Berlin, Germany

Francisco A. Sylvester, MD (Question 20)
Professor of Pediatrics and Immunology
Connecticut Children's Medical Center
University of Connecticut Health Center
Hartford, Connecticut

Jonathan E. Teitelbaum, MD (Question 36)
Director of Pediatric Gastroenterology
The Children's Hospital at Monmouth
    Medical Center
Long Branch, New Jersey
Associate Professor of Pediatrics
Drexel University School of Medicine
Philadelphia, Pennsylvania

Charles P.B. Vanderpool, MD (Question 3)
Assistant Professor of Clinical Pediatrics
Pediatric Gastroenterology, Hepatology,
    and Nutrition
Riley Hospital for Children at Indiana
    University Health
Indianapolis, Indiana

*Narayanan Venkatasubramani, MBBS, MD
    (Question 25)*
Assistant Professor
Department of Pediatrics
Duke University Medical Center
Durham, North Carolina

Dascha C. Weir, MD (Question 30)
Division of Gastroenterology and
    Nutrition
Boston Children's Hospital Harvard
    Medical School
Boston, Massachusetts

Steven L. Werlin, MD (Question 25)
Professor
Medical College of Wisconsin
Milwaukee, Wisconsin

Keith E. Williams, PhD (Question 6)
Professor of Pediatrics
Director of Pediatric Feeding Program
Penn State Hershey Children's Hospital
Hershey, Pennsylvania

Harland Winter, MD (Question 37)
Director, Pediatric Inflammatory Bowel
   Disease
MassGeneral Hospital for Children
Boston, Massachusetts

Nader N. Youssef, MD (Question 11)
Digestive Health Care Center
Senior Medical Director
GI Clinical Development
NPS Pharmaceuticals
Bedminster, New Jersey

Bella Zeisler, MD (Question 41)
Division of Digestive Diseases,
   Hepatology and Nutrition
Connecticut Children's Medical Center
Assistant Professor of Pediatrics
University of Connecticut School of
   Medicine
Hartford, Connecticut

Foreword

The field of pediatric gastroenterology has expanded dramatically in the last 20 years. Indeed, many pediatricians, family physicians, and other health care providers now feel the need for an up-to-date, readable, and reliable guide to our field. This volume is ideally suited to that purpose; it contains answers to the 49 most commonly asked questions in pediatric gastroenterology in succinct and focused, practice-directed mini-chapters. This book will not only provide some pearls, but also make you look good.

The book is brief enough that it can be read cover to cover, but for physicians who wish to look up a specific question, both the table of contents and index are easily accessible. Topics cover a broad range of information. If you want the latest approach to colic, it is here. If you need help for your patients with constipation and incontinence, it is here. If you want to know when to request a consultation with a pediatric gastroenterologist, you will find that information here in a concise disease-related fashion. If you are looking for ways in which to synergize your practice with that of your consulting gastroenterologists, they are here. If you need details about screening for neonatal liver disease and other important hepatic disorders, they are here. From the common to the rare disorders, information will guide your decision making.

In the process of using this guide in your office (I suggest keeping it close at hand in your exam room[s]; in fact you may want more than one copy!) you will not only become a source of new management strategies, but you will also feel confident in your advice. I cannot recommend this volume strongly enough. I hope you enjoy it as much as I have.

Richard J. Grand, MD
Professor of Pediatrics
Harvard Medical School Director Emeritus
Center for Inflammatory Bowel Disease Program Director Emeritus
Clinical and Translational Study Unit
Children's Hospital Boston Division of Gastroenterology and Nutrition
Brookline, Massachusetts

Introduction

"If I had more time, I would have written you a shorter letter."

—Abraham Lincoln

It is undeniably true that our world runs at a faster pace than that of our 16th president. So while letters may have been better crafted in President Lincoln's day, all our communications are now much more rapid. In our fast-paced days as medical care providers, we all experience times when we would love to have a few minutes with a master clinician or researcher to help us quickly understand a patient's problem and find an answer for them. *Curbside Consultations* is designed to give you such an opportunity. We have lined up a panel of experts in pediatric gastroenterology and have posed 49 pressing and common clinical questions to them. Their answers are brief, and we think you will agree they are very impactful. In just a few pages, each question is answered by one of the most pre-eminent authorities in the field. Using an easy and almost conversational style, our experts provide the knowledge, insight, and all the clinical pearls you will need to be able to tackle the clinical issue at hand. We hope you find this format both helpful and practical—enjoy!

SECTION I

COMMON PROBLEMS
IN INFANCY

HOW IS INFANT COLIC DIAGNOSED AND TREATED?

Audra S. Rouster, MD and Paul E. Hyman, MD

Infant colic is defined using Wessel's rule of 3s as the following: crying for more than 3 hours per day, at least 3 days per week, for at least 3 weeks, in an infant who is otherwise growing and developing normally.[1] Although there is a strict definition, you should identify infant colic whenever crying exceeds a caregiver's ability to cope with an otherwise healthy infant. Colic typically starts around 2 weeks of age and peaks at 6 weeks of age.[2] By 12 weeks of age, 60% of infant colic resolves and by 16 weeks of age 90% resolves. Premature infants follow the predicted course based on their due date and not their chronological age. Colic occurs in roughly 20% of all infants. There is no association with gender, ethnicity, socio-economic status, feeding preference, or birth order.

Crying episodes associated with colic have a clear start and end with no association to the events leading up to the episode; they are not predictable. The worst episodes often occur in the evening. Efforts to soothe the infant seem futile, although they may lessen the intensity of the crying. Infants may draw up their legs, develop an abdomen that is firm to the touch, and become flushed. The constellation of a crying infant and the abdomen appearing tense causes some caregivers to assume that the infant is experiencing abdominal pain. There are no data to support a view that an infant experiencing colic is in pain, although there are also no data disproving it either. Many caregivers will describe their baby as excessively gassy, prompting referral to a gastroenterologist. All infants swallow air, more so when they are crying. When screaming, infants increase intra-abdominal pressure, so flatus passes. Explaining that the gassiness is a result of the excessive crying, and not the cause, may make conservative measures seem more reasonable to the caregiver. If the crying episodes start after the 3rd month or persist beyond the 4th month, then a re-evaluation is warranted.

To diagnose colic you should obtain a history from the caregiver. While the caregiver is watching, complete a thorough physical exam. It is reassuring to the caregiver if you point out normal and healthy findings, including growth parameters graphed on a chart.

Treatment for colic should focus on education, support, and reassurance for the caregivers. By the time the infant is brought to a specialist's office, most families have already tried many remedies without avail. Many products have been studied, both pharmaceutical and homeopathic. With several, the risks outweigh the absence of benefit: anticholinergic drugs such as dicyclomine,[3] gripe water (its contents are not regulated by the Food and Drug Adminstration), and herbal teas (these pose a risk of hyponatremia and inadequate caloric intake). Other ineffective but not harmful interventions include simethecone,[3] probiotics, and lactose-free diets.[3]

Two medical interventions are worth trying. If the infant is fed with cow or soy protein formula, consider a 2-week trial of a hydrolyzed protein formula.[1] Typical signs or symptoms of a milk protein allergy include emesis, blood in the stool, diarrhea, eczema, failure-to-thrive, and colicky abdominal pain. Explain to the caregiver the Rule of Ones, that is if the only symptom is intractable fussing without any of the above signs and symptoms, than the diagnosis is infant colic. However, if there is intractable fussiness and any one of the other symptoms listed above, treat the formula protein allergy by changing to hydrolyzed protein formula. The infant should return to the initial formula if no improvement is noted.[4] Additional formula changes are not necessary or desirable. Amino acid-based formulas have not been shown to have any additional benefit beyond a protein hydrolysate. If the mother is breastfeeding, a 2-week trial eliminating cow milk and soy products from her diet would be the equivalent; there is no need to stop breastfeeding.

The second medical intervention is to educate about and treat infant regurgitation if there is frequent spitting-up.[1] Infant regurgitation, defined as infants who spit up 2 or more times a day for 3 weeks or longer, is a functional disorder found in about 50% of all healthy infants. Treatment for infant regurgitation includes thickening the formula with cereal, feeding only to satiety, and positioning the head upright after meals. Infant regurgitation resolves spontaneously by the end of the first year. Unless there is gastroesophageal reflux disease defined by food refusal and failure to gain weight, blood in stool or emesis, or chronic or acute lung disease, no acid suppressing medications are needed.

It is reassuring to the caregiver for you to re-evaluate the infant frequently, even weekly, in your office. It comforts the caregiver when you do a physical exam and the infant is plotted on the growth chart. Being able to observe the caregiver/infant interaction is vital. Screening caregivers regularly for depression is appropriate, and you provide support and encouragement at each visit. Anyone who has ever had a baby or even seen a baby will be offering the caregiver advice on how to make the crying stop. You should educate the caregiver about how there are no known treatments for curing colic but also no long-term adverse outcomes. Colic resolves over time without medical intervention.

Nonmedical interventions are encouraged, because they allow the caregiver active participation in the treatment of the infant. Maneuvers such as swaddling the infant tightly, providing non-nutrient sucking with a pacifier, and white noise may help. Motion is another intervention; taking the infant for a car ride, placing the infant in a swing or a bouncy seat that vibrates, even seating the infant in the car seat on the washing machine as it cycles are all ways that might soothe the infant. Infants responding to these maneuvers reassure caregivers that the crying is not caused by pain, because what kind of pain responds to a car ride?

The most important piece of information for you to share with the caregiver is that he or she is not alone. Unconsciously, caregivers may resent the infant with colic. Caregivers feel obliged to love the infant unconditionally, but a screaming infant who is unresponsive to their soothing efforts provokes many negative thoughts and emotions. There is social pressure placed on caregivers to be competent to comfort their own infant. You must be sure to convey understanding for both the spoken and unspoken needs of the caregiver, including the need for respite care and rallying a strong support system. Colicky infants are at a higher risk of shaken baby syndrome.[5] Caregivers should hold their infant and attempt soothing maneuvers but if they begin to feel frustrated, they should not feel guilty about placing the infant in a safe place, such as the crib, for 10 to 15 minutes while they do something to soothe themselves.

References

1. Drossman DA, Corazziari E, Delvaux M, et al. *Rome III: The Functional Gastrointestinal Disorders.* 3rd ed. McLean, VA: Degnon Associates; 2006:699-703.
2. Fireman L. Colic. *Pediatr Rev.* 2006;27(9):357-358.

3. Lucassen PL, Assendelft WJ, Gubbels W, van Eijk TM, van Geldrop WJ, Knuistingh Neven A. Effectiveness of treatments for infantile colic: systematic review. *BMJ*. 1998;316:1563-1569.
4. American Academy of Pediatric Committee on Nutrition. Hypoallergenic formulas. *Pediatrics*. 2000;106:346-349.
5. Fujiwara T, Barr RG, Brant R, Barr M. Infant distress at five weeks of age and caregiver frustration. *J Pediatr*. 2011;159: 425-430.

WHAT ARE THE CAUSES OF
RECTAL BLEEDING IN INFANTS?

Natalie Sikka, MD and Ian Leibowitz, MD

Finding blood in the diaper in an otherwise healthy infant is a common clinical presentation, accounting for as much as 10% of referrals to pediatric gastroenterologists in some studies. While generally not reflecting a complex underlying diagnosis, bleeding is extremely scary to parents and warrants an initial evaluation focused on assessing whether the infant has a common source, such as a perianal fissure or a rarer but more serious condition such as intussusception. Table 2-1 provides a list of the etiologies (common and uncommon) of bright-red rectal bleeding during infancy.

As with many diagnoses in infants, listening to the history from the parents is critical. Has the child been feeding poorly, had colicky episodes, or periods of lethargy? Was the formula changed recently, has the mother been on antibiotics while breastfeeding, or have the stools been hard?

A perfectly happy, healthy, thriving child is certainly more likely to have a perianal fissure, whereas a baby with poor feeding or periods of pain or vomiting may be of greater concern to have an intussusception or other anatomic lesion. Do not forget that infants with intussusception are frequently more lethargic and "septic" in appearance as opposed to older children who often present with episodes of colicky pain. It is important to identify the timeline of bleeding and any associated signs, symptoms, or events. An infant with bloody diarrhea after antibiotics may warrant stool tests, especially for *Clostridium difficile*, recognizing that many infants may be colonized by this organism but become symptomatic after antibiotics. Streaks of blood that have been present for several days in an otherwise healthy infant most likely represent a protein-induced proctocolitis, to be discussed later.

A physical exam that includes seeing the stool or getting a detailed description of the bleeding is the next step in evaluating the possibilities. Is the blood bright red or maroon colored, with the stool or by itself, mixed with mucous or just on the wipe after cleaning? The physical exam needs to address not only looking for signs of obstruction in the abdomen but also the overall status of the child. A sick-appearing child could have a volvulus, necrotizing enterocolitis, or an infection. These children rarely present with isolated rectal bleeding and often will also have a history of vomiting or abdominal distension and abnormal physical exam. Such conditions need rapid attention. Large amounts of blood without stool or darker bleeding may suggest a vascular or anatomic cause and warrant aggressive evaluation. Once evaluation has ruled out the serious considerations that require immediate intervention, a large group of otherwise healthy infants with bleeding

---

Table 2-1
Etiologies of Bright-Red Rectal Bleeding During Infancy

- Protein-induced proctocolitis
- Coagulopathy
- Duplication cyst
- Hirschsprung enterocolitis
- Infectious colitis
- Intestinal duplication
- Intussusception
- Lymphonodular hyperplasia
- Malrotation with volvulus
- Meckel's diverticulum
- Necrotizing enterocolitis
- Perianal fissure
- Vascular malformation

---

remains. The 2 most common causes of rectal bleeding in these infants are perianal fissures and protein-induced proctocolitis. The infants with these conditions are usually gaining weight, growing, and developing appropriately. They typically present with streaks or dots of blood in the diaper or on the stool.

Perianal fissures are frequently seen as a result of the passage of a hard stool, though they can occur in the absence of a clear constipation history. Bleeding almost always is limited to the end of the stooling process, either on the wipe or the end of a formed stool. Fissures can be seen on physical exam but are often missed if there is an incomplete effort to spread the gluteal muscles apart to enable full visualization. Making the effort to get a good exam may spare children further evaluation. Topical creams and ointments may be helpful in healing external irritation. If stools are persistently hard, recommending a few ounces of prune juice, or baby prunes in older infants, may provide relief. If there is still no difference, consider the possibility of food intolerance as the cause of the hard stools. It is not uncommon for food intolerance, most commonly cow's milk protein and soy protein intolerance, to manifest as constipation. In these children, hypoallergenic formulas frequently result in stools that are extremely loose and relieve the constipation. Finally, there are infants who continue to have hard stools in spite of dietary changes (eg, those requiring cereal added to their formula); these infants may actually benefit from small doses of stool softeners like lactulose on a daily basis.

Protein-induced proctocolitis is another common cause of rectal bleeding. As most of these conditions are non-immunoglobulin E (IgE) mediated, they are usually referred to as intolerances, hence the common usage of the term *cow's milk protein intolerance* (CMPI). These infants are generally healthy and thriving though a subgroup will present with significant diarrhea and failure to thrive in conjunction with their bleeding. Recognizing which babies have self-limited proctocolitis from those with a more diffuse enteropathy is the first challenge. As a general rule, good weight gain and no change in the character of the stooling (ie, increase in frequency or change to watery diarrhea) other than the presence of blood and perhaps mucus, defines the milder form of this condition. A child with poor weight gain and more profuse diarrhea may have a true enterocolitis and warrants a more aggressive approach. Both variants typically result from sensitivity to cow's milk protein or soy protein and can occur in breastfed or formula fed infants. There is good evidence that maternal ingestion of cow's milk protein leads to its presence in breast milk and absorption by the infant.

Unfortunately, there is no single diagnostic test for these protein sensitivities, so empiric elimination of the suspected agent is frequently the next step. If an infant is breastfed, the mother will need to exclude the protein from her diet that generally begins with elimination of all sources of cow's milk protein. As many patients with CMPI will cross react to soy proteins because of their significant homology, many physicians recommend avoiding soy as well. If the child is thriving, a step-wise approach may be easier on the mother. In formula fed infants, casein hydrosylate formulas are generally recommended, as about 80% of the cow's milk proteins are caseins in nature. Trials of these formulas or an elimination diet should occur for at least 14 to 21 days before considering them a failure (recovery of the mucosal inflammation after removal of an immunologic stimulus may take time). In formula fed children who do not respond or in those with a more serious enteropathy with anemia, hypoalbuminemia, and weight loss, an amino acid-based formula may be appropriate. For breastfed infants, we find it helpful to present the options to the parents (ie, while mother is eliminating the allergen from her diet, she may continue to breastfeed through the bleeding or "pump and save" while using a partially hydrolyzed or elemental formula). It is important to provide parents with a list of what to look for on ingredient labels. In the case of cow's milk protein elimination, it is important to educate parents on the difference between lactose and milk protein. Many individuals believe that lactose-free products are allowed, whereas most lactose-free products do contain milk protein.

If there is no appreciable difference in the rectal bleeding after the elimination of cow's milk protein and soy protein from the mother's diet, you may consider elimination of the other more common food allergens (ie, eggs, wheat, and nuts). However, we recommend elimination of one food at a time and emphasize the importance of attention to the nutritional adequacy of the mother's diet. A mother who has eliminated most protein and fat sources from her diet will not be providing nutritionally complete breastmilk to her infant.

There is variation in the approach to treating protein-induced proctocolitis. Some practitioners will tolerate the occasional streak of blood, whereas some will want to see complete resolution, including hemoccult negative stool samples. We believe that the occasional streak of blood is tolerable, with the caveat that an increase in the amount of blood warrants a complete blood count and coagulation profile with further evaluation as indicated. The limited natural history data suggest mild cases will resolve without complication. If the diagnosis is in doubt, a flexible sigmoidoscopy with biopsies may be indicated. Visual inspection of the mucosa in patients with protein-induced proctocolitis may demonstrate erythema, hemorrhagic erosion, and/or lymphonodular hyperplasia. Biopsies may demonstrate eosinophilic infiltrate.

There are very little data to guide the timing of reintroduction of the sensitizing protein. If cow's milk protein and soy protein are not tolerated, we recommend the use of a partially hydrolyzed or elemental toddler formula and continued reintroduction of the allergen every few months. The prognosis of protein-induced proctocolitis is quite good, with most children tolerating a regular diet within the first 2 years of life and only a minority developing a true allergy.

Recently, attention has been given to the possible relationship between disruption of intestinal microbiota and rectal bleeding in those infants with presumed protein-induced proctocolitis. There are data supporting the use of *Lactobacillus GG* along with a partially hydrolyzed formula as being more helpful than the use of a partially hydrolyzed formula alone. Accordingly, some companies are adding probiotics to their infant formulas.

This discussion has focused on how to evaluate the infant with bright red blood per rectum, with further elaboration on the 2 most common causes (perianal fissures and protein-induced proctocolitis). While rectal bleeding is a common presenting symptom to pediatricians, most infants will fortunately not have serious underlying diagnoses. A rapid evaluation to rule out threatening anatomic, infectious, and vascular anomalies will generally lead the pediatrician to consideration of the common causes discussed previously.

Bibliography

Arvola T, Ruuska T, Keranen J, Hyöty H, Salminen S, Isolauri E. Rectal bleeding in infancy: clinical, allergological, and microbiological examination. *Pediatrics*. 2006;117(4):e760-e768.

Baldassarre M, Laforgia N, Fanelli M, Laneve A, Grosso R, Lifschitz C. *Lactobacillus* GG improves recovery in infants with blood in the stools and presumptive allergic colitis compared with extensively hydrolyzed formula alone. *J Pediatr*. 2010;156(3):397-401.

Kay M, Wyllie R. Gastrointestinal hemorrhage. In: Wyllie R, Hyams JS, eds. *Pediatric Gastrointestinal and Liver Disease: Pathophysiology, Diagnosis, Management*. Philadelphia, PA: Saunders; 2006:203-215.

Turck D, Michaud L. Lower gastrointestinal bleeding. In: Walker WA, et al, eds. *Pediatric Gastrointestinal Disease: Pathophysiology, Diagnosis, Management*. Hamilton, Ontario, Canada: BC Decker Incorporated; 2004:266-280.

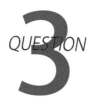

How Is Gastroesophageal Reflux Disease Diagnosed in Infants and What Are the Best Treatments?

Charles P.B. Vanderpool, MD and
Sandeep Gupta, MD, AGAF, FACG, FASGE, FAAP

Gastroesophageal reflux (GER) is defined as the involuntary passage of gastric contents into the esophagus. Gastroesophageal reflux disease, or GERD, occurs when GER causes complications or worrisome symptoms. It is important to note that physiologic GER occurs multiple times per day in otherwise healthy infants, children, and adults, though there are a variety of protective mechanisms that prevent esophageal mucosal damage. Failure of these mechanisms can lead to symptoms and signs associated with GERD (Table 3-1). The diagnostic and therapeutic approach to GER/GERD in an infant should be tailored to address the concerns that lead to the caregiver seeking medical attention, focused initially on history and physical examination.

The diagnosis of GER/GERD is often made by history and physical examination, though symptoms and signs associated with GER in infants may be nonspecific (see Table 3-1). Frequent regurgitation, irritability, and vomiting can occur in infants with physiologic GER or GERD and can also be associated with alternative diagnoses such as food intolerance/allergy or infantile colic. Despite these drawbacks, history and physical examination are paramount in attempting to determine if more worrisome disorders may be present, as well as weighing the risks and benefits of empiric treatment versus those of further diagnostic testing. Following a complete and detailed history and physical examination, we will offer only parental reassurance and support if physiologic GER is suspected as pharmacological therapy has not been shown to alter the course of physiologic GER.

If further testing is warranted, evaluation may include an upper gastrointestinal (GI) contrast study, nuclear scintigraphy, esophagogastroduodenoscopy (EGD) with biopsies, or 24-hour continuous intra-esophageal pH monitoring study ("pH probe") with or without impedance monitoring (Table 3-2). While readily available, an upper GI study should not be used for the routine diagnosis of GER or suspected GERD in infants. An upper GI study is performed over a brief duration of time, leading to frequent false-positive results for the occurrence of GER and over-interpretation of normal physiologic reflux episodes. Considering these limitations, we use the upper GI study as a tool to evaluate for anatomic abnormalities, such as esophageal web or

Table 3-1
Signs and Symptoms in Infants That May Be Related to Gastroesophageal Reflux Disease

Symptoms	Signs
Regurgitation	Sandifer syndrome (dystonic neck posturing)
Vomiting	Recurrent pneumonia
Poor weight gain	Apnea spells
Irritability	Feeding refusal
Wheezing	Sleeping disturbances
Cough	
Persistent hiccups	

Table 3-2
Diagnostic Studies Useful in Infant Gastroesophageal Reflux Disease and Typical Indication

Study	Indication
Upper GI contrast radiography	Suspected anatomic abnormality includes esophageal web or stenosis, tracheoesophageal fistula, hiatal hernia, antral web, pyloric stenosis, and malrotation
	Symptoms include severe feeding refusal, immediate or projectile vomiting, and bilious vomiting
Gastroesophageal nuclear scintigraphy	Evaluation for reflux and pulmonary aspiration
	Negative test does not preclude intermittent pulmonary aspiration
Esophageal pH monitoring with/ without impedance	Determine if episodic symptoms are related to esophageal reflux
	Often used when pulmonary/airway symptoms present
Upper GI endoscopy	Evaluate worrisome sign/symptom or alternative diagnosis
	Symptoms include feeding refusal, dysphagia, failure to thrive, and no improvement following therapy

stricture, tracheoesophageal fistula, hiatal hernia, antral web, pyloric stenosis, and intestinal malrotation (see Table 3-2).

Gastroesophageal nuclear scintigraphy is performed using ingestion of food labeled with the radioisotope ⁹⁹technetium. A device capable of detecting the signal emitted by this radioisotope is then used to obtain intermittent images of the stomach and esophagus to evaluate for GER. Nuclear scintigraphy can also provide information regarding gastric emptying time that may be prolonged in infants or children with gastric dysmotility accompanying GERD. Similar to upper GI studies, nuclear scintigraphy may not differentiate between physiologic and pathologic GER. Unlike an upper GI study, nuclear scintigraphy can offer the benefit of evaluating if GER is associated with pulmonary aspiration in infants with persistent respiratory symptoms. If secondary aspiration is suspected, delayed images up to 24 hours later should be requested. It is important to realize that a negative test does not preclude infrequent or intermittent pulmonary aspiration (see Table 3-2).

Commercially available pH probe systems for infants include a catheter for transnasal insertion into the distal esophagus and a system to capture and analyze episodes of acidic reflux into the esophagus. A drop in the esophageal pH < 4.0 is considered an acid-reflux episode; the percentage of time during a 24-hour study that the esophageal pH is < 4.0 constitutes the reflux index (RI) and is the most commonly used summary score. An abnormal RI, however, has not been shown to consistently correlate with GERD symptom severity or the presence of esophagitis in infants. Esophageal electrical impedance monitoring in addition to pH monitoring has recently been suggested as an additional tool in the evaluation of GER/GERD in infants. It detects changes in electrical impedance caused when a bolus of fluid or air passes between electrical sensors along a nasally inserted catheter. Esophageal pH monitoring with or without impedance measurement may be used in instances where episodic symptoms are thought to be related to GER (see Table 3-2). We may use impedance monitoring when pulmonary or airway symptoms are thought to be related to GER, as it detects both acidic and nonacidic episodes of GER. Unfortunately, the true predictive value of these measurements in establishing a casual relation between specific symptoms and GER has not been consistently established in pediatrics studies. Impedance measurements and pH have also failed to reliably predict infants who may benefit from anti-reflux surgery. As a result, their usefulness in the diagnosis and management of GERD in infants is limited to select situations as determined within centers with expertise in these studies.

EGD serves an important role in select situations in the evaluation of GERD in infants. It allows direct visual examination and biopsy of the upper GI tract, recognizing that normal macro- and/or microscopic findings do not rule out nonerosive GERD. We typically reserve EGD to evaluate concerning symptoms and signs in infants, such as acute or severe feeding refusal, dysphagia, failure to gain weight, or lack of clinical improvement with conservative therapy or pharmacological interventions (see Table 3-2). Diagnoses that can be investigated during endoscopy include esophageal stricture or web, hiatal hernia, antral web, and other causes of esophagitis, including infectious esophagitis, caustic ingestion, or eosinophilic esophagitis. This procedure often requires administration of general anesthesia and should be performed in centers with expertise in pediatric endoscopy.

As symptoms of GERD in infants can be nonspecific and there is no single test that can clearly diagnose pathologic GERD in all patients, infants are often treated presumptively with anti-reflux medical therapy. However, the approach to treatment of GERD should be based on the presenting symptoms, their severity, and the presence or absence of complications related to these symptoms. Management options include lifestyle changes, dietary modifications, pharmacological therapy, and anti-reflux surgery (Table 3-3). In infants, lifestyle changes include avoidance of over-feeding, offering less volume of feeds but at frequent intervals, burping during and after feeds, limited movement following feeds, and avoidance of exposure to tobacco smoke. A variety of nutritional interventions may be considered; a subset of infants with a intolerance or allergy to cow's milk protein may experience symptoms of regurgitation and vomiting similar to physiologic GER.

Table 3-3

Treatment Options for Gastroesophageal Reflux Disease in Infants (Includes Non-Food and Drug Administration/ Off-Label Use)

Treatment	Description
Lifestyle/nutritional modification	Anti-reflux precautions
	Limited trial of hydrolyzed formula
	Dietary elimination of milk protein from breastfeeding mother
	Addition of thickening agent
Acid-suppressive therapy	H2RAs include ranitidine, famotidine, and nizatidine
	PPIs include omeprazole, lansoprazole, and esomeprazole
Prokinetic therapy	Erythromycin, metoclopramide (black box warning), and bethanechol
Surgical therapy	Fundoplication is typically reserved for significant GERD-related complications (eg, aspiration and pneumonia)

Studies support a trial for up to 4 weeks of an extensively hydrolyzed or free amino acid formula in infants with excessive vomiting or regurgitation. In human-milk fed infants, we may also consider elimination of cow's milk protein from the mother's diet; however, symptoms are rarely severe enough to warrant cessation of human milk. Other dietary interventions include the addition of thickening agents such as infant rice cereal; infant oatmeal cereal may be used instead in the setting of concomitant constipation. Thickening the formula does not decrease the RI measured during pH studies, but may decrease the frequency of visible regurgitation. We utilize up to 1 tablespoon of infant cereal per 2 ounces of standard 20 kilocalorie per ounce (kcal/oz) formula. It is important to realize that 1 tablespoon of rice cereal contains approximately 14 kcal; thus 1 tablespoon of rice cereal per 2 ounces of 20 kcal/oz formula increases the formula's caloric density to approximately 27 kcal/oz. The caloric density of cereal should be confirmed based on the brand and amount utilized for thickening. Commercially available antiregurgitant formulas retain the standard 20 kcal/oz concentration when mixed, according to the manufacturer's direction and may also lead to a slight decrease in visible regurgitation. Noncereal thickening agents are also available commercially. Nipple size may need to be increased to allow free-flow of formula during feeding.

Pharmacologic interventions include acid-suppressive therapy and prokinetic agents (see Table 3-3). Acid-suppressive therapy in infants is largely limited to H2-receptor antagonists (H2RA) and proton pump inhibitors (PPI). Rapid-acting oral antacids, such as magnesium and aluminum compounds, should not be used in infants due to the lack of clear dosing guidelines and potential toxicity associated with these medications. In infants with concerning symptoms consistent with GERD, an initial trial of H2RA therapy is appropriate and may include ranitidine, famotidine, or nizatidine. We typically do not utilize cimetidine due to its less favorable side effect profile, including a slight risk of hepatic and endocrine side effects. The long-term efficacy of H2RA therapy is limited by tachyphylaxis; diminution of response may occur within 6 weeks of therapy. PPIs have been shown to have superior efficacy in healing of erosive esophagitis, and their efficacy does not diminish with chronic use. PPIs that are currently approved in North America for use in children include omeprazole, lansoprazole, and esomeprazole. Oral formulations of these medications have yet to achieve the Food and Drug Administration approval in infants. Studies in infants with GERD-like symptoms have failed to show superiority of PPI when compared to placebo in symptom improvement despite documented acid control. Increasing evidence suggests that acid suppression associated with H2RAs or PPIs may increase the rates of lower respiratory tract infections (including pneumonia) and gastroenteritis in infants and children. Acid suppression, especially to the degree seen with PPI use, should thus be used with caution in this age group and if used should be directed at a specific symptom or complication, be used for a defined period of time, and should be monitored under consistent physician observation.

The physiology of infantile GER would suggest early use of prokinetic therapy. Studies have shown an improvement in RI with use of prokinetic agents including cisapride and metoclopramide. However, use of both of these medications is limited by their side effect profile. Cisapride is no longer routinely available in the United States due to concerns regarding prolongation of the QTc interval of the cardiac cycle, as measured on a standard electrocardiogram. Metoclopramide commonly results in adverse side effects in infants, including lethargy, irritability, and gynecomastia. Metoclopramide also carries a significant risk of extrapyramidal reactions, including permanent tardive dyskinesia and now carries a black box warning regarding this risk. Given this, we will typically utilize prokinetic therapy in patients who have documented gastroparesis or when delayed gastric emptying is highly suspected. Erythromycin does improve gastric emptying, but its use in infants with GER or GERD has not been well established, and it is associated with risks of developing pyloric stenosis if used in the first few weeks of life. Bethanechol, a cholinergic agonist, may be considered in infants with GERD but side effects, including complication of respiratory issues such as reactive airway disease, limit its use in infants.

Surgical therapy consisting of fundoplication is typically reserved for infants who have significant complications related to GERD, including secondary aspiration and aspiration pneumonia (see Table 3-3). Infants with neurologic disability, cardiac disease, or other comorbidities with significant GERD are more likely to be considered for fundoplication. The majority of patients who undergo fundoplication have improvement in the degree of reflux and regurgitation with fewer GERD-related complications. Side effects from fundoplication can be common and may include retching, bloating, and accelerated gastric emptying. Additionally, the fundoplication may break down or fail over time.

Conclusion

Physiologic GER is common in infants and frequently does not require diagnostic evaluation or treatment in otherwise healthy infants. Parental support and reassurance is often sufficient in these cases. When pathologic GERD is suspected, diagnostic evaluation should be directed at the most concerning symptom(s) and may include radiographic studies, endoscopic evaluation, or esophageal pH monitoring. The decision to pursue diagnostic evaluation may be weighed against the risks and benefits of presumptive therapy. When therapy with acid suppression is utilized, it should typically be done within a defined time frame and not be continued indefinitely unless clearly indicated based on a more extensive evaluation.

Bibliography

Rudolph CD, Hassall E. Gastroesophageal reflux. In: Kleinman RE, Sanderson IR, Goulet O, Sherman PM, Mieli-Vergani G, Shneider BL, eds. *Walker's Pediatric Gastrointestinal Disease.* 5th ed. Hamilton, Ontario, Canada: BC Decker Inc; 2008:59-71.

Vandenplas Y. Gastroesophageal reflux. In: Wyllie R, Hyams JS, eds. *Pediatric Gastrointestinal and Liver Disease, Pathophysiology/Diagnosis/Management.* 3rd ed. Philadelphia, PA: Saunders; 2006:305-325.

Vandenplas Y, Rudolph CD, Di Lorenzo C, et al. Pediatric Gastroesophageal Reflux Clinical Practice Guidelines: Joint Recommendations of the North American Society for Pediatric Gastroenterology, Hepatology, and Nutrition (NASPGHAN) and the European Society for Pediatric Gastroenterology, Hepatology, and Nutrition (ESPGHAN). *J Pediatr Gastroenterol Nutr.* 2009;49(4):498-547.

WHAT IS THE NORMAL STOOLING PATTERN FOR AN INFANT AND WHAT MEDICATIONS CAN I SAFELY USE FOR A CONSTIPATED INFANT?

Silvana Bonilla, MD and Alejandro F. Flores, MD

An infant's stooling pattern is different from the stooling pattern of toddlers and older children. A baby's first bowel movement (meconium) is sticky in consistency and greenish to black in color. The characteristics of the stool change as the infant grows; stools turn yellow, green, or brown in color and consistency is either formed or unformed. Frequency also transitions from high (more than 4 stools per day) in infants to 1 stool per day in toddlers aged 4 years. The frequency and consistency of stools vary from infant to infant and depend mostly on the food the infant is being fed. Breastfed infants generally have 3 or more soft to runny stools a day, usually after feedings. These infants rarely develop hard stools that are difficult to pass. In some instances, the frequency of stools may be lower than the average, which does not necessarily indicate that the infant is constipated. Infants that are fed formula may have fewer stools when compared to breastfed infants.

Observational studies conducted in a primary care setting have shown that up to 3% of infants developed constipation in the first year of life. Symptoms frequently present at the time of transition from breast milk to cow's milk-based formulas or when the infant starts eating solids. Some clinical manifestations include irritability, grunting, poor tolerance of feedings, arching of the back, and stiffening of the legs. Parents sometimes interpret these symptoms as if the infant is straining to defecate. In infants younger than 6 months, you should also consider other conditions such as infant dyschezia. This condition is characterized by excessive straining and crying with defecation followed by successful passage of soft to liquid stools. Intervention is usually not necessary and symptoms improve with time.

Diagnostic criteria for constipation in infants and toddlers younger than 4 years have been suggested (Table 4-1). These symptom-based criteria, also known as Rome criteria, were developed as a tool to facilitate the diagnosis of childhood functional gastrointestinal disorders. If the child meets the criteria, you can be reassured that the likely origin of symptoms is nonorganic. However, there are some special situations in which you have to pay extra attention since the likelihood of a serious condition increases. One example is constipation presenting in the newborn or early in life. Failure to pass meconium during the first 48 hours of life is highly suggestive of organic conditions, such as Hirschsprung's disease (HD) (Table 4-2). A comprehensive history and physical

Table 4-1
The Rome III Criteria for Functional Constipation in Neonates and Toddlers

At least 2 of the following symptoms must occur for at least 1 month:
- Less than 2 defecations per week
- More than one episode per week of incontinence after the acquisition of toileting skills
- History of excessive stool retention
- History of painful or hard bowel movements
- Presence of a large fecal mass in the rectum
- History of large-diameter stools that may obstruct the toilet

Table 4-2
Organic Etiologies of Constipation in Infants

- Endocrine
  - Hypothyroidism
  - Diabetes
- Metabolic
  - Hypercalcemia
  - Hypokalemia
- Congenital
  - HD
- Toxins
  - Lead poisoning
- Medications
  - Over-the-counter cold medication
  - Antacids
  - Codeine
- Genetic
  - Cystic fibrosis
- Neurologic
  - Cerebral palsy
  - Spinal cord problems (eg, myelomeningocele)

Table 4-3

Medications to Be Considered in the Treatment of Constipation in Infants Older Than 1 Month

Polyethylene glycol (MiraLax)	0.4 g/kg body weight per day or 0.7 g/kg body weight/day
Lactulose or sorbitol	(10 g/15 mL) 1 to 3 mL/kg body weight/day, divided in 1 to 2 doses
Milk of magnesia	1 to 3 mL/kg body weight/day, divide in 1 to 2 doses

examination with attention to the abdominal exam, anal inspection, rectal digital examination, and perianal sensation testing (anal wink), will help you rule out anatomical defects of the ano-rectal area, such as anal atresia, anal stenosis, or an abnormally placed anus. Spinal defects such as myelomeningocele must also be ruled out by physical exam, and if needed, further imaging studies should be obtained. Rare congenital conditions such as HD should be considered. HD is characterized by the absence of ganglion cells in the submucosal and myenteric plexus that are responsible for the motility of the large intestine. Diagnostic work-up for this condition includes a barium enema, anorectal manometry, and possibly a rectal suction biopsy. Meconium plugs, which are sometimes associated with cystic fibrosis, are also a consideration in the differential for infant constipation. Other organic causes of constipation include endocrine, metabolic, and neurological conditions.

Management of infant constipation should start with parental education. You should take time to provide an explanation for the symptoms to the parents as well as debunk frequent myths. The different interventions used to treat constipation share the same goal, which is to alleviate or resolve painful defecation and associated symptoms such as abdominal pain or fecal soiling. Dietary modifications are usually the first line of treatment. The addition of small amounts of high-sugar–containing foods to the infant's diet, such as juices (ie, prune, pear, and apple) or corn syrup and offering pureed fruits and vegetables is sometimes sufficient to improve symptoms. For formula-fed infants, changing formulas might sometimes lead to clinical improvement. On average, 1 in 4 infants improve with these recommendations. In infants that fail to improve, you may consider the use of osmotic laxatives. Agents that are associated with an excellent safety profile and response in this age group include polyethylene glycol, lactulose, sorbitol, or milk of magnesia (magnesium hydroxide). The effective dose of these medications in this particular age group is variable. Suggested doses based on available literature are listed in Table 4-3. The dose can be titrated up or down from the starting dose to achieve optimal results.

Conclusion

The stooling pattern of infants differs from infant to infant and is strongly related to the infant's diet. Constipation is not uncommon in infants and it usually presents when there are changes in the diet, such as the introduction of formula or solid foods. Most of the time behavioral factors and voluntary withholding are involved in the generation of symptoms. Dietary modifications are the first line of treatment followed by osmotic laxatives that lead to the resolution of symptoms in most of the cases. In special cases, such as in infants presenting with symptoms in the neonatal period or not responding to proper treatment, we consider further evaluation to rule out potential organic etiologies.

Bibliography

Hyman PE, Milla PJ, Benninga MA, Davidson GP, Fleisher DF, Taminiau J. Childhood functional gastrointestinal disorders: neonate/toddler. *Gastroenterology.* 2006;130(5):1519-1526.

Loening-Baucke V. Prevalence rates for constipation, feacal and urinary incontinence. *Arch Dis Child.* 2007; 92:486-489.

Loening-Baucke V, Krishna R, Pashankar DS. Polyethylene glycol 3350 without electrolytes for the treatment of functional constipation in infants and toddlers. *J Pediatr Gastroenterol Nutr.* 2004;39:536-539.

Loening-Baucke V, Pashankar DS. A randomized, prospective, comparison study of polyethylene glycol 3350 without electrolytes and milk of magnesia in children with constipation and fecal incontinence. *Pediatrics.* 2006;118:528-535.

Nurko S, Youssef NN, Sabri M, et al. PEG3350 in the treatment of childhood constipation: a multicenter, double-blinded, placebo-controlled trial. *J Pediatr.* 2008;153:254-261.

REFLUX AND VOMITING IN INFANTS ARE SO COMMON, WHEN SHOULD I SEND AN INFANT FOR EVALUATION ESPECIALLY TO EXCLUDE ANATOMIC AND METABOLIC DISEASES?

Colin Rudolph, MD, PhD

Gastroesophageal reflux (GER) is a normal physiologic event that describes the passage of stomach contents into the esophagus, and sometimes from the mouth. This is usually referred to as regurgitation, spitting-up, or poseting in infants. Episodes of GER can be quite forceful, which can make it difficult to discriminate physiologic (normal) reflux from vomiting. Episodes of regurgitation in infants are usually effortless and the child is otherwise happy and comfortable. GER is more common following a meal since distension of the stomach triggers the relaxation of the lower esophageal sphincter, allowing venting of the stomach as occurs with burping. The infant with uncomplicated GER is often referred to as a "happy spitter" since the gastric contents are extruded from the mouth but the infant is not distressed. This occurs in half of normal infants at least one time per day; with 20% having more than 4 episodes per day until 6 months of age. The frequency decreases after 6 months of age such that by 12 months of age, regurgitation is uncommon, although intermittent episodes may occur following large meals or with activity until about 18 months of age.

Vomiting is a coordinated reflex that is triggered by a region of the brainstem in response to noxious stimuli, including gastrointestinal (GI) inflammation, toxins, or vestibular stimuli. Activation of this reflex stimulates episodes of retroperistalsis in the upper GI tract with expulsion of upper GI contents from the mouth. In contrast to GER, vomiting is usually associated with the uncomfortable sensation of nausea characterized by pallor, seating, and retching. Although infants and young children are unable to verbally describe the feeling of a "need to vomit," they do demonstrate the signs associated with vomiting and generally appear distressed.

When to Worry?

Despite this difference in the underlying mechanisms of GER versus vomiting, discriminating between the 2 can be difficult even for the experienced clinician. Therefore, a symptom-based management approach that does not discriminate between these has been recommended.[1]

Table 5-1

Warning Signals and Referral in the Infant With Reflux or Vomiting

Urgent or emergent evaluation (the acutely unwell infant)	Bilious or forceful vomiting
	Hematemasis and/or hematochezia
	Abdominal distension and/or tenderness
	Alterations in mental status or seizures
	Apnea/acute life-threatening events
	Fever associated with vomiting
	Diarrhea with dehydration
	New onset hepatosplenomegaly with vomiting
	Acute onset of feeding refusal, odynophagia, and dysphagia
Requires further evaluation (the otherwise well infant)	Onset or increase in vomiting after 6 months of age
	Growth failure
	Recurrent pneumonia/wheezing
	Chronic irritability or discomfort
	Feeding refusal, odynophagia, dysphagia, or discomfort during feeding
	Atopy or a family history of atopy
	Developmental delay, macrocephaly, and micro-cephaly
	Upper airway symptoms

A careful history and physical exam helps determine when further evaluation is warranted. Exclusion of warning signals establishes a diagnosis of "uncomplicated GER" in an otherwise well infant. Wellness implies that the infant is happy, gaining weight and height appropriately, and achieving normal developmental milestones. Warning signals that warrant immediate evaluation versus those that may require referral for less urgent evaluation are listed in Table 5-1. Causes of vomiting are listed in Table 5-2. It is beyond the scope of this chapter to describe the approach to evaluate each symptom or sign.

Acute changes in a previously well infant, such as bilious vomiting, abdominal tenderness or distension, the new onset of vomiting associated with fever, or a change in mental status warrant emergent evaluation. In these situations, vomiting is usually one of a constellation of symptoms and signs that guide further directed urgent or emergent evaluation and/or referral. Bilious vomiting with or without abdominal tenderness and distension may be associated with GI obstruction. Bilious vomiting can occur with severe vomiting that is not due to obstruction but in all situations emergent evaluation is required due to the possibility of malrotation with volvulus. Other surgical

Table 5-2
Causes of Vomiting

GI obstruction	Pyloric stenosis
	Malrotation
	Antral web
	Incarcerated hernia
	Foreign body
Neurologic	Hydrocephalus
	Subdural hematoma
	Mass lesion
	Intracranial hemorrhage
Infectious	Sepsis
	UTI
	Pneumonia
	Otitis media
	Hepatitis
	Meningitis
Metabolic/endocrine	Diabetes mellitus
	Galactosemia
	Hereditary fructose intolerance
	Urea cycle defects
	Amino/organic acidemias
	Congenital adrenal hyperplasia
Renal	Obstructive uropathy
	Renal insufficiency
Toxic	Lead
	Iron
	Vitamin A and D toxicity
	Medications

(continued)

emergencies, such as neonatal appendicitis, torsion of an ovary or testis, or incarcerated hernia may also present with abdominal distension or tenderness. Nonbilious, forceful vomiting may be due to pyloric stenosis. Vomiting with hematemesis or hematochezia may occur with these surgical disorders or may result from erosive esophagitis, or mucosal inflammation such as peptic ulcer disease. It may also be caused by a foreign body with mucosal erosion, prolapse gastropathy, or a Mallory-Weiss tear (barotrauma to the gastric mucosa due to forceful retching). Generally,

Table 5-2 (continued)
Causes of Vomiting

Cardiac	*Congestive Heart Failure*
Other GI	Achalasia
	Gastroparesis
	Gastroenteritis
	Peptic ulcer
	Food allergy
	Eosinophilic esopahgitis
	Inflammatory bowel disease
	Pancreatitis
	Appendicitis

hematemesis or hematochezia warrant urgent endoscopic evaluation if surgical disorders are not suspected. The new onset or increased severity of vomiting associated with fever is often a sign of infections including sepsis, meningitis, urinary tract infection, otitis media, or infectious diarrhea. Vomiting associated with mental status changes also requires emergent evaluation since it may result from neurologic disorders, such as a subdural hematoma or intracranial hemorrhage, or with metabolic and endocrine disorders, such as urea cycle disorders or congenital adrenal hyperplasia. Toxin exposures may also present with acute vomiting, often with associated mental status changes or seizure. Apnea or acute-life threatening events are typically not due to GER but require urgent evaluation to rule out neurologic, cardiac, and airway disorders.

In an infant with frequent regurgitation or chronic vomiting, further evaluation should also be considered if the infant has a new onset of vomiting, increased frequency, or increased severity of vomiting after 6 months of age. It is important to be aware that normal physiologic reflux often increases in frequency between 2 and 6 months of age and therefore, below the age of 6 months, an increase in frequency without other warning signals is not worrisome. GER is rarely the cause of growth failure unless meal volume is restricted in an effort to prevent regurgitation. In such cases, parental education about a normal GER and diet counseling may be helpful, but further evaluation to determine the cause of growth failure is generally required. If poor growth persists, disorders including infections (especially urinary tract during infancy), food allergy, anatomic abnormalities, neurologic disorders, metabolic disease, and neglect or abuse should be considered.

Unexplained crying irritability may be due to esophagitis, but other causes such as infant colic, food allergy, neurologic disease, or infection need to be considered. Empiric therapy with proton pump inhibitors (PPIs) has not been shown to be effective.[2] Prior to treating possible esophagitis, a trial of a hydrolyzed protein formula may be considered. In infants with atopy or a family history of atopy, recurrent vomiting is more likely to be due to food allergy or eosinophilic esophagitis. Upper endoscopy will differentiate between infectious esophagitis, eosinophilic esophagitis, or reflux esophagitis providing guidance for therapy if esophagitis is present.

Dysphagia, odynophaia, or food refusal can result from reflux esophagitis. However, other causes, including a foreign body, eosinophilic esophagitis, and neurologic disorders may also cause these symptoms. Following a careful neurologic evaluation, referral for an esophagram and/or upper GI endoscopy is recommended. Dystonic posturing may be due to GER (Sandifer syndrome), but evaluation by a neurologist is generally indicated.

Older children (aged 8 to 10 years and older) are able to reliably describe heartburn. In such cases, empiric therapy with either an H2-blocker or PPI is reasonable. If the child improves, continued therapy for up to 3 months is reasonable. If symptoms recur following discontinuing therapy or if symptoms persist despite treatment, referral to a pediatric gastroenterologist should be considered.

Respiratory complications that are often attributed to GER include acute life-threatening events (ALTEs), wheezing, and reactive airway disease. ALTEs may be associated with infection, child abuse, upper airway obstruction, cardiac, respiratory, metabolic, and neurologic disorders. In the vast majority of infants, GER is not the cause of ALTEs so other etiologies must be considered. GER is one of the causes of recurrent pneumonia particularly in high-risk children, including those with poor airway protection due to neurologic disease or anatomic disorders of the airway or esophagus. Prior to considering GER as causative, other causes, including immunodeficiency, cardiac disease, and pulmonary anatomic disorders, should be ruled out. Recurrent wheezing or asthma has been purported to be exacerbated by GER. However, medical therapy with PPIs has not been demonstrated to be efficacious in treatment of pediatric asthma.[3] Therefore, if an infant or child has recurrent asthma or wheezing, a referral for further evaluation to rule out airway disease or to optimize asthma management should be considered. Chronic hoarseness and other laryngeal disorders have also been attributed to gastroesophageal reflux disease, but evidence of improvement with proton pump therapy in infants, children, and adults is lacking. Since other disorders need to be ruled, referral for laryngoscopy should be considered.

References

1. Vandenplas Y, Rudolph CD, Di Lorenzo C, et al. North American Society for Pediatric Gastroenterology Hepatology and Nutrition, European Society for Pediatric Gastroenterology Hepatology and Nutrition. Pediatric gastroesophageal reflux clinical practice guidelines: joint recommendations of the North American Society for Pediatric Gastroenterology, Hepatology, and Nutrition (NASPGHAN) and the European Society for Pediatric Gastroenterology, Hepatology, and Nutrition (ESPGHAN). *J Pediatr Gastroenterol Nutr.* 2009;49(4):498-547.
2. Orenstein SR, Hassall E, Furmaga-Jablonska W et al. Multicenter, double-blind, placebo-controlled trail assessing the efficacy and safety of proton pump inhibitor lansoprazole in infants with symptoms of gastroesophageal reflux disease. *J Pediatr.* 2009;154:514-520.
3. Writing Committee for the American Lung Association Asthma Clinical Research Centers. Holbrook JT, Wise RA, Gold BD, et al. Lansoprazole for children with poorly controlled asthma: a randomized controlled trial. *JAMA.* 2012;307(4):373–381.

WHY DO SOME INFANTS FEED POORLY AND WHAT INTERVENTIONS ARE BEST FOR THESE INFANTS AND THEIR PARENTS?

Douglas G. Field, MD and Keith E. Williams, PhD

In normal infant feeding, satiety and comfort reinforce regular cycles of hunger and successful eating. However in some infants, this cycle is disrupted or may never develop. For parents, the feeding of one's infant can be a rewarding experience, but for parents of children who exhibit feeding problems, it can be a frustrating and stressful experience.

Feeding problems are nonspecific in newborns and young infants. A large number of medical conditions have been demonstrated to be related to pediatric feeding problems and some of these are summarized in Table 6-1. Such medical conditions may make eating difficult, uncomfortable, or even painful.[1] As a result, the infant's motivation to eat is decreased. Additionally, there are commonly used medications that can cause nausea, irritability, or decreased appetite. Out of sheer desperation to have their child eat, parents may take actions, such as feeding during an infant's sleep, allowing the child to have a bottle or drink at any time, or avoiding novel foods that the child may initially refuse. These parental reactions may maintain or even worsen the child's feeding problem.

Feeding problems are common in infants and most often are transient and do not adversely affect growth and development. Predisposing conditions include prematurity especially with a history of bronchopulmonary dysplasia and mechanical ventilation. Infants with hypotonia, static encephalopathy, and other neurologic compromise may also develop chronic feeding problems. These feeding problems can include slow feeding, vomiting while eating, gagging or choking on food or drink, difficulty transitioning to table food, limited intake, dysphagia or difficulty with swallowing, and refusal to eat. An evaluation of these problems consists of several components, including a feeding history, medical history, physical examination, feeding observation, and medical testing.

Feeding history focuses on the following questions:
- When did the feeding problem begin?
- Is this an acquired or congenital problem?
- Is the child breastfed, bottle fed, or tube dependent?

Table 6-1
Medical Conditions Associated With Feeding Problems

Anatomic abnormalities	Naso-oropharyngeal problems can include choanal atresia, cleft lip or palate, ankyloglossia, macroglossia, and Pierre Robin sequence
	Laryngeal problems can include laryngeal cleft, subglottic stenosis, laryngeal cyst, and laryngo-tracheomalacia
	Esophageal structural problems include tracheoesophageal fistula, congenital esophageal stenosis, vascular rings, esophageal stricture, esophageal foreign body, and achalasia
Neurodevelopmental problems	CP, familial dysautonomia, muscular dystrophies, myasthenia gravis, myelomeningocele, seizures, and Arnold-Chiari malformation
Cardiopulmonary problems	Congenital heart disease, bronchopulmonary dysplasia, and asthma
GI problems	GER, EE, delayed gastric emptying, food allergies, and esophageal foreign body

GI: gastrointestinal; CP: cerebral palsy; GER: gastroesophageal reflux; EE: eosinophilic esophagitis.

- If bottle fed, what type and amount of formula does the child consume?
- What types, textures, and amounts of solid foods does the infant eat?
- How long is a typical meal?
- Does the child show evidence of food aversion such as crying, mouth clenching, head turning, or throwing food?

The goal of the feeding history is to determine not only what the child is eating, but how the child is being fed. This information will be critical in helping to develop feeding recommendations for the family.

A detailed medical history may give some indication of the etiology of the child's feeding problem. Aspiration should be suspected in infants with recurrent pneumonias, wheezing or coughing, or gagging with feeds. Vomiting, irritability, arching with feeds, or diarrhea may suggest gastroesophageal reflux disease (GERD) or possibly a cow's milk protein allergy.[2] Stridor may represent subglottic stenosis or other upper airway abnormality. Dysphagia, vomiting, or drooling may represent a gastrointestinal (GI) anatomic abnormality, such as esophageal atresia or stricture, gastric outlet obstruction, pyloric stenosis, or intestinal malrotation.

The physical examination begins with the measurement of weight, height, and head circumference, and this information should be followed longitudinally at each visit. Poor growth usually results from inadequate caloric intake, but it could also be indicative of malabsorption or a medical condition causing increased caloric expenditure. Craniofacial abnormalities (ie, cleft lip, cleft palate, macroglossia, and ankyloglossia) and signs of systemic disease (ie, wheezing, cardiac murmur, clubbing, cyanosis, and eczema) should be identified.

A feeding observation should assess the child's positioning during feeding, interactions with the caregiver, and oral motor skills. Such an evaluation will help with intervention planning and may allow medical problems to be uncovered. For example, discoordination of sucking/swallowing/breathing may suggest choanal atresia, increased congestion across the meal may indicate aspiration, and vomiting later in the meal may be the result of a motility or anatomic abnormality. This observation may be conducted by the physician or by therapists experienced in the treatment of infant and pediatric feeding problems.

While medical testing is not required for all children, laboratory studies should be performed in children who have evidence of poor growth. These studies include complete blood count, sedimentation rate, albumin, hepatic and renal function, thyroid function tests, total IgA level, and tissue transglutaminase antibody. Fecal fat to assess for fat malabsorption and sweat chloride test to evaluate for cystic fibrosis can be performed. An upper GI series can be done in infants with vomiting or dysphagia to assess upper GI anatomy. An esophagogastroduodenoscopy can help to assess for mucosal abnormalities from reflux or EE.

The outlined feeding assessment will direct the development of a planned intervention. For example, if a food allergy is demonstrated, exclusion of allergenic foods (eg, milk, soy, eggs, nuts, wheat, and fish) from the maternal diet of breastfed infants and the use of a hypoallergenic formula in bottle fed infants is indicated. For children who have already moved to complimentary foods, nutritional counseling may help the family maintain an allergy-free diet. If GER is diagnosed, treatment can be instituted (see Question 34).

While medical management of associated and predisposing medical conditions is important, it often does not resolve the feeding issue. The treatment plan should include nutritional recommendations, especially if there are special diets required such as in the case of food allergies or other underlying medical conditions. For infants having difficulty with weight gain, caloric intake can be increased by concentrating formulas or adding powdered formula to breast milk. Solid foods can be fortified with butter, vegetable oil, powdered milk, or glucose polymers. If these methods of calorie enhancement are not sufficient, supplemental feeding via nasogastric tube or gastrostomy tube feedings may need to be considered.

Since infants or toddlers with feeding issues may have conditioned aversions to eating and may not express hunger well, treatment also involves modifications to the feeding environment. Most importantly, the caregivers need to be trained to utilize well formulated feeding structure. A schedule of meals and snacks, typically 4 to 6 per day, is recommended. The child should be fed in the same place, in order to help the child develop a hunger-satiety cycle. We also recommend these feedings be time limited, lasting no longer than 15 to 20 minutes. It is common to see families who feed their child multiple times across the day or who feed for prolonged periods of time, in some cases in excess of an hour. In our clinical experience, this is not helpful. For infants who are extremely irritable during feedings, minimizing stimulation such as feeding in a quiet room or swaddling the infant may be of benefit. If an infant is difficult to arouse, gentle massage may stimulate the infant enough to result in better feeding. Parents should to be taught how to recognize an infant's hunger and satiety cues, avoid overfeeding, and minimize distractions during meal time.

For children who are having difficulty eating solid foods, there are several effective behavioral interventions. One of these interventions, stimulus fading, involves systematic changes to the food or liquid.[3] This can be accomplished in many ways. For children who have trouble increasing texture, fading has been used to slowly increase the texture of the foods presented so the child can adapt to the texture without gagging or refusal. For children who drink formula but refuse water or milk, fading has been used to increase acceptance of the target liquid. In this case, small amounts of formula are systematically replaced with the target liquid, until the child is drinking only the target liquid without formula. Because fading involves making only small changes over time, it is often easy for parents to use and well accepted by the children. Since children with feeding problems may demonstrate little internal motivation to eat either because of a lack of appetite or conditioned aversions, other interventions involving external motivation in the form of positive reinforcement can be employed.

Reinforcement-based interventions often involve providing the child with access to videos, favorite toys, and other preferred objects or activities. This can be effective in cases where the child exhibits a feeding behavior such as eating a specific number of bites. We often tell parents that reinforcement is a helpful tool that can be used to improve eating until the child finally finds the food itself to be reinforcing. In addition to teaching parents to reinforce appropriate eating behavior, we teach parents to ignore inappropriate behaviors such as crying, throwing food, or gagging.

There are a variety of resources available for patients with feeding problems. Many hospitals have feeding programs or clinics staffed with speech pathologists, occupational therapists, nutritionists, psychologists, and/or other providers who specialize in working with children with feeding problems. Early intervention programs can also provide therapists who can help with feeding issues. Pediatric medical subspecialists, especially pediatric gastroenterologists, can help manage the medical and nutritional needs of these children.

References

1. Kedesdy JH, Budd PS, eds. *Childhood Feeding Disorders: Biobehavioral Assessment and Intervention.* Baltimore, MD: Paul H. Brookes Publishing Co; 1998.
2. Haas AM, Maune NC. Clinical presentation of feeding dysfunction in children with eosinophilic gastrointestinal disease. *Immunol Allergy Clin North Am.* 2009;29(1):65-75.
3. Williams KE, Foxx RM. *Treating Eating Problems in Children With Autism Spectrum Disorders and Developmental Disabilities.* Austin, TX: Pro-Ed; 2007.

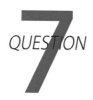

QUESTION

7

How Long Do I Follow a Newborn With Prolonged Jaundice and How Much Work-Up Should I Do Before Sending the Child to a Specialist?

Henry Lin, MD and David A. Piccoli, MD

Neonatal jaundice is a common pediatric problem with approximately 50% of term and up to 80% of preterm infants developing jaundice in the first week of life. Most instances of neonatal jaundice are benign and few infants have significant underlying disease. The challenge for clinicians is to determine when further evaluation is needed.

Jaundice is a yellowing of the skin and mucous membranes that is caused by the deposition of bilirubin. Bilirubin is the end product of heme-protein catabolism. This bilirubin is unconjugated and insoluble. Unconjugated bilirubin is conjugated in the liver by uridine diphosphoglucuronic acid—glucuronyl transferase into a soluble form for excretion in the bile. Neonatal jaundice can result from accumulation of either type of bilirubin and distinguishing between conjugated or unconjugated bilirubin is important in determining the etiology of hyperbilirubinemia and neonatal jaundice.

There are 2 measurement systems for bilirubin. The usual assay measures the "direct" reacting and total bilirubin with indirect bilirubin being a calculated measurement. A limitation of this assay is that infants with physiologic jaundice can have an abnormal elevated "direct" fraction that is not actually conjugated bilirubin. The other bilirubin assay independently measures total bilirubin, conjugated bilirubin, and unconjugated bilirubin. A delta fraction, which represents bilirubin covalently bound to albumin, is also calculated.

Almost all neonatal jaundice that occurs in the first week of life is due to unconjugated bilirubin. Unconjugated hyperbilirubinemia is defined as a total serum bilirubin level above 5 mg/dL and most commonly is a result of neonatal physiology. Physiologic jaundice occurs in up to 15% of newborns and is due to increased bilirubin production that primarily results from relative polycythemia and increased red blood cell turnover in neonates. Newborns produce 6 to 8 mg/kg of bilirubin per day, which is twice the adult rate. Bilirubin production typically declines to adult levels within 2 weeks after birth, thus accounting for the self-resolution of physiologic jaundice. Breastfeeding increases the likelihood of jaundice and should be considered as an etiology.

Table 7-1

Causes of Unconjugated Hyperbilirubinemia

Overproduction

- Hemolytic
  - ABO or minor blood group incompatibility
  - Fetal hydrops
  - Spherocytosis
  - Elliptocytosis
  - G6PD deficiency
  - Pyruvate kinase deficiency
  - Hemoglobinopathy
  - Infections
- Nonhemolytic
  - Physiologic
  - Breastfeeding jaundice
  - Birth trauma (eg, cephalohematoma, intraventricular hemorrhage, and swallowed blood)
  - Polycythemia
  - Pyloric stenosis
  - Cystic fibrosis
  - Ileal atresia

Decreased Conjugation

- Prematurity
- Breast milk jaundice
- Hypothyroidism
- Gilbert syndrome
- Crigler-Najjar syndrome

The causes of neonatal unconjugated hyperbilirubinemia can be classified by mechanism as either overproduction or decreased conjugation of bilirubin. Overproduction of bilirubin can further be subdivided into hemolytic and nonhemolytic causes (Table 7-1). Specific etiologies include extravasated blood, hemolytic disease, erythrocyte membrane defects, erythrocyte enzyme deficiencies, inborn errors of metabolism, and increased enterohepatic circulation from pyloric stenosis or obstruction. Diagnosis is aimed at the exclusion of these conditions. Prolonged, asymptomatic mild elevation of unconjugated bilirubin should suggest a disorder of bilirubin conjugation such as Gilbert's syndrome. For the most part, neonatal unconjugated hyperbilirubinemia does not require subspecialty consultation. Treatment is directed toward the underlying cause. For physiologic jaundice, phototherapy and rarely, exchange transfusion, have been used to help with bilirubin excretion. The purpose of treatment is to prevent kernicterus, which results from deposition of bilirubin in the brain.

While most neonatal jaundice results from deposition of unconjugated bilirubin, conjugated hyperbilirubinemia in infancy is a relative emergency that requires prompt evaluation. In the neonate, many cholestatic liver diseases present with conjugated hyperbilirubinemia. Cholestasis is physiologically defined as a reduction in bile flow from the liver and is clinically characterized by the accumulation of substances that are normally excreted in bile (cholesterol, bile acids, and bilirubin). Bile flow is dependent on bile acid secretion, while bilirubin is processed by a separate conjugation and transport mechanism. Therefore, an infant may be cholestatic without being jaundiced.

Conjugated hyperbilirubinemia affects 1 in 2500 infants and should be suspected when jaundice persists beyond 2 weeks of life. Specifically, conjugated hyperbilirubinemia is defined as a conjugated fraction of bilirubin either greater than 2 mg/dL or 15% of an abnormal total bilirubin level. Determining the cause of conjugated hyperbilirubinemia requires several diagnostic tests. The majority of the evaluation is focused on the concern of cholestatic diseases, in particular on biliary atresia where the outcome and treatment are time sensitive. In general, once a neonate is noted to have conjugated hyperbilirubinemia beyond 2 weeks of life, the neonate should be referred to a pediatric gastroenterologist.

A variety of disorders present with cholestasis during the neonatal period. Newborns are at an increased risk for these disorders due to a combination of immature hepatic excretory function, increased susceptibility to infection, and the presentation of the initial effects of congenital malformations and inborn errors of metabolism during this time period. The etiology of conjugated hyperbilirubnemia can be classified by area of involvement: extrahepatic biliary disease, intrahepatic biliary disease, and hepatocellular disease (Table 7-2). The differential diagnosis of conjugated hyperbilirubinemia depends on the clinical situation and should be guided by the initial physical exam and laboratory studies. The initial work-up should be focused on conditions that are most amenable to treatment, which include etiologies such as sepsis, urosepsis, galactosemia, tyrosinemia, hypothyroidism, and structural diseases, specifically biliary atresia.

Biliary atresia is a progressive fibro-obliterative disease of unclear etiology that is due to destruction of the extrahepatic biliary tree. Most cases of biliary atresia are isolated to the liver and hepatobiliary tree, but 15% to 20% of biliary atresia is associated with other congenital malformations. There is an insidious onset of jaundice as infants with biliary atresia tend to look well. Treatment is surgical with the creation of a Kasai hepatoportoenterostomy that allows for drainage of the biliary tree from the porta hepatis into a roux limb of the bowel. The goal of a Kasai is to reduce the chance of liver transplantation. The outcome of a Kasai is directly correlated to the child's age at the time of operation, thus reflecting the urgency of diagnosis. Aside from biliary atresia, other common etiologies of neonatal cholestasis include idiopathic neonatal hepatitis, alpha-1-antitrypsin deficiency, inherited syndromes, and TORCHES (toxoplasmosis, other infections, rubella, cytomegalovirus, herpes simplex) infections.

Clinical findings in neonatal conjugated hyperbilirubinemia are independent of etiology and do not differentiate between types of disease. Commonly reported clinical findings include acholic stools, jaundice, scleral icterus, and dark urine. The physical exam should focus on identifying known causes of pathological jaundice and involves assessment for evidence of dehydration, extravasated blood, pallor, petechiae, and hepatosplenomegaly. Other findings may include ascites, portal hypertension, lethargy, growth failure, xanthomas, and heme-positive stools. It has been suggested that serum bilirubin can be estimated by the level of jaundice on the body. Unfortunately, this is not a consistently reliable estimation. The correlation between jaundice and serum bilirubin levels is unreliable once jaundice extends below the middle of the chest.

Table 7-2
Causes of Conjugated Hyperbilirubinemia

Extrahepatic Biliary Disease
- Structural disease
  - Biliary atresia
  - Choledochal cyst
  - Choledocholithiasis
  - Neoplasm

Intrinsic Biliary Disease
- Syndromes
  - Alagille syndrome
  - Caroli disease
  - Congenital hepatic fibrosis
  - Nonsyndromic paucity of bile ducts
  - Polysplenia syndrome (heterotaxy)
  - Inspissated bile syndrome

Hepatocellular Disease
- Drugs/toxins
  - Parenteral nutrition
- Infectious
- Bacterial
  - Gram negative sepsis
  - Syphilis
  - Toxoplasmosis
  - UTI/pyelonephritis
- Viral
  - Coxackievirus B
  - Cytomegalovirus
  - Echovirus
  - HBV
  - Herpesvirus
  - HIV
  - Rubella virus

(continued)

<u>Table 7-2 (continued)</u>
Causes of Conjugated Hyperbilirubinemia

- Inherited non-cholestatic jaundice syndromes
    - Dubin-Johnson syndrome
    - Rotor syndrome

Metabolic

- Amino acid pathways
    - Tyrosinemia
- Sugar metabolism pathways
    - Galactosemia
    - Hereditary fructose intolerance
    - Other metabolic inherited disorders
- Syndromes
    - Turner syndrome
    - Trisomy 17, 18, or 21
    - Zellweger syndrome
- Bile salt and transport abnormalities
    - Aagenaes syndrome (recurrent cholestasis with lymphedema)
    - Benign familial recurrent cholestasis
    - Bile acid synthesis defects
    - FIC1
    - BSEP
    - MDR3

Systemic Disease

- Congestive heart failure
- Generalized hemangiomatosis
- Hypopituitarism
- Postnecrotizing enterocolitis
- Postshock or postasphyxia

UTI: urinary tract infection; HBV: hepatitis B virus; HIV: human immunodeficiency virus; FIC1: PFIC 1 familial intrahepatic cholestasis-1; BSEP: PFIC 2 bile salt export pump deficiency; MDR3: PFIC 3 multidrug resistance protein 3 deficiency.

The history and physical exam findings should guide the work-up process and the initial evaluation depends on the age of the newborn. Typical initial assessment should focus on general hematologic, liver, and infectious studies. The conjugated hyperbilirubinemia should be confirmed via a total and conjugated bilirubin level. A complete blood count with differential, reticulocyte count, and peripheral smear should be obtained to evaluate for sepsis and hemolysis. Assessment of liver function should include transaminases, alkaline phosphatase, and gamma-glutamyl transpeptidase. Synthetic liver function should be evaluated via prothrombin time, international normalized ratio, albumin, and serum cholesterol level. Urine studies should be obtained to rule out infection, galactosemia, and renal Fanconi syndrome via a urinalysis and urine succinylacetone. Other infectious etiologies should also be assessed via blood cultures and TORCHES infection titers. If no obvious etiology is found, radiograph studies as well as additional serologic studies should be considered in addition to a referral to a pediatric gastroenterologist.

Abdominal ultrasound with Doppler can help with evaluation of the biliary tree especially if the gallbladder is not visualized on a fasting ultrasound. For further evaluation of biliary anatomy, a radionuclide scan can be performed. The radionuclide tracer is normally taken up by the hepatocytes and secreted into the bile. Nonexcretion of the radionuclide into the intestine 24 hours after injection should be concerning for biliary obstruction or hepatocellular dysfunction. If radiologic studies do not reveal an etiology, a percutaneous liver biopsy should be considered. Specifically, the biopsy can help with the diagnosis of biliary atresia. In the absence of biliary obstruction, a liver biopsy can distinguish among other causes such as Alagille syndrome, alpha-1 antitrypsin deficiency, and infectious etiologies. Of note, in early biliary atresia, a liver biopsy may be indistinguishable from hepatitis and ultimately require a repeat biopsy.

Overall, neonatal jaundice is a clinical manifestation of a diverse range of disorders. Jaundice that persists for more than 2 weeks in a formula-fed infant or 3 weeks in a breast-fed infant requires additional evaluation. Conjugated hyperbilirubinemia is never physiologic and should prompt immediate evaluation. Referral to a pediatric gastroenterologist is essential if the etiology remains unknown or if the jaundice remains prolonged. Treatment of neonatal jaundice is based on the underlying disease.[1-6]

References

1. Suchy FJ. Approach to the infant with cholestasis. In: Suchy FJ, Sokol RJ, Balistreri WF, eds. *Liver Disease in Children*. 3rd ed. Cambridge, UK: Cambridge Univeristy Press; 2007:179-189.
2. Evans D. Neonatal jaundice. *Clin Evid (Online)*. 2007:pii:0319.
3. Jatla M, Haber BA. Jaundice. In: Liacouras C, Piccolo D, eds. *Pediatric Gastroenterology: The Requisites in Pediatrics*. Philadelphia, PA: Mosby. 2008:276-284.
4. Porter ML, Dennis BL. Hyperbilirubinemia in the term newborn. *Am Fam Physician*. 2002;65(4):599–606.
5. Moyer V, Freese DK, Whitington PF, et al. North American Society for Pediatric Gastroenterology, Hepatology and Nutrition. Guideline for the evaluation of cholestatic jaundice in infants: recommendations of the North American Society for Pediatric Gastroenterology, Hepatology and Nutrition. *J Pediatr Gastroenterol Nutr*. 2004;39(2):115–128.
6. American Academy of Pediatrics Subcommittee on Hyperbilirubinemia. Management of hyperbilirubinemia in the newborn infant 35 or more weeks of gestation. *Pediatrics*. 2004;114(1):297-316.

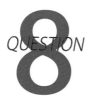
WHAT IS THE CORRECT MANAGEMENT AND FOLLOW-UP FOR INFANTS WHOSE MOTHERS ARE INFECTED WITH HEPATITIS B?

Douglas Mogul, MD, MPH and Kathleen B. Schwarz, MD

In the United States, the incidence of acute hepatitis B virus (HBV) infection in children younger than 15 years has declined by 98% from 1990 to 2006. This decrease can be attributed both to the introduction of the universal infant vaccination in 1991, as well as recommendations for the use of hepatitis B immunoglobulin (HBIG) in neonates born to HBsAg (hepatitis B surface antigen)-positive mothers.[1,2] However, while the incidence of HBV infection is declining, approximately 24,000 HBV-infected women give birth each year in the United States.[3] Furthermore, neonates are especially susceptible to developing chronic hepatitis B (CHB) as compared to older children and adults. While only 5% to 10% of acutely infected adolescents and adults will develop CHB, 90% of neonates and 25% to 50% of children aged 1 to 5 years will develop CHB.[4] The younger the age of acquisition, the higher the risk of cirrhosis, liver failure, and hepatocellular cancer.[4] Clearly, aggressive monitoring of the immunization status of pregnant women as well as a comprehensive vaccine strategy for newborns has been a successful public health intervention and ongoing vigilance is necessary.

The correct management and follow-up for infants whose mothers are infected with hepatitis B hinges on what is known about the maternal HBV status, as well as the infant's birth weight. The American Academy of Pediatrics (AAP), as well as the Advisory Committee for Immunization Practices (ACIP) from the Centers for Disease Control (CDC) have established guidelines for immunoprophylaxis, and these guidelines were recently supported in a consensus statement from pediatric hepatologists.[4-6] All neonates born to HBsAg-positive mothers should receive a dose of the monovalent HBV vaccine of 0.5 mL IM and HBIG 0.5 ml IM at 2 different injection sites within 12 hours of delivery (Table 8-1). Furthermore, infants with a birth weight less than 2.0 kg will require an additional dose of the vaccine at 2 to 3 months as part of their series; therefore, such infants receive vaccine within 12 hours of delivery, and 1 month, 2 to 3 months, and 6 to 7 months. If the HBsAg status of the mother is unknown, then an infant with birth weight greater than 2.0 kg should receive the recombinant vaccine and the mother's HBsAg status should be tested immediately. Should the mother be subsequently found to be HBsAg-positive, then the infant must receive HBIG within 7 days of life. At the same time, an infant less than 2.0 kg who is born to a mother with unknown HBsAg status should receive HBIG provided this information

Table 8-1

Guidelines for the Passive and Active Immunoprophylaxis Against Hepatitis B Virus for Term and Low Birth Weight Infants

Maternal HBsAg Status	*Infant Birth Weight ≥ 2000 g*	*Infant Birth Weight < 2000 g*
Positive	Hepatitis B vaccine and HBIG, both within 12 hrs of birth 3 vaccine doses at 0, 1, and 6 months of chronological age Check anti-HBs and HBsAg at 9 to 15 months; if infant is HBsAg and anti-HBs negative, reimmunize with 3 doses at 2-month intervals and retest	Hepatitis B vaccine and HBIG, both within 12 hrs of birth 4 vaccine doses at 0, 1, 2 to 3, and 6 to 7 months of chronological age Check anti-HBs and HBsAg at 9 to 15 months; if infant is HBsAg and anti-HBs negative, reimmunize with 3 doses at 2-month intervals and retest
Unknown	Hepatitis B vaccine within 12 hrs of birth Test HBsAg in mother; if HBsAg-positive, give HBIG within 7 days and follow additional guidelines for infants born to HBsAg-positive mothers	Hepatitis B vaccine within 12 hrs of birth Test HBsAg in mother immediately; if results are unavailable by 12 hrs, or if HBsAg-positive, then give HBIG and follow additional guidelines for infants born to HBsAg-positive mothers
Negative	3 vaccine doses at 0, 1 to 2 months, and 6 to 18 months	First dose of hepatitis B vaccine at 30 days of chronological age if medically stable, or at hospital discharge Second and third doses of vaccine at 2 to 4 and 6 to 18 months, respectively

Adapted from Saari TN. Immunization of preterm and low birth weight infants. American Academy of Pediatrics Committee on Infectious Diseases. *Pediatrics.* 2003;112(1 pt 1):193-198.

is not available by 12 hours of life. If the mother is ultimately found to be HBsAg-positive, these infants will require a fourth dose of the vaccine to complete their series. Lastly, it should be noted that infants less than 2.0 kg born to HBsAg-negative mothers should not receive their first dose until 30 days of life, or at hospital discharge if less than 30 days old. However, these infants will only need 3 doses to insure adequate immunogenicity with the second dose to be given at 2 to 4 months and the final dose at 6 to 18 months.

For those children born to HBsAg-positive mothers, postvaccination monitoring is an important part of their follow-up. We agree with the CDC and ACIP recommendations that children born to infected mothers should be screened for HBsAg and anti-HBs at 9 to 18 months in order to demonstrate that the child did not get infected and that he or she had an appropriate response to the recombinant vaccine. It is important to wait until 9 months of age to adequately demonstrate that anti-HBs is the result of active immunization and not circulating anti-HBs from the HBIG. By 9 months, it can be assumed that children who are anti-HBs have developed a durable response to HBV. Children who are negative for HBsAg and anti-HBs should receive a second series of the vaccine (3 doses, each 2 months apart) and again be screened to evaluate their response to the re-immunization. Finally, children who are persistently positive for HBsAg represent the 5% to 10% of children for which active and passive immunoprophylaxis fail, likely secondary to intrauterine transmission and/or perinatal acquisition by infants born to mothers with a high viral load.[7] Children with persistent HbsAg positive status should be referred to a pediatric hepatologist.

At present, alpha-interferon is the only anti-viral therapy that is approved by the Food and Drug Administration (FDA) for children as young as 1 year; it should not be given to children younger than this because of the risk of spastic diplegia.[8] Other therapies that are FDA approved for patients in the pediatric age group are lamivudine starting at 2 years, adefovir (starting age 12 years), and entecavir (starting age 16 years). These therapies are described in detail in Jonas et al.[9] Trials in young children are currently underway for entecavir and pegylated alpha-interferon.

One frequent question the general pediatrician or neonatologist gets asked is whether it is safe for a mother with HBV to breastfeed a newborn. Although HBV has been detected in breast milk, studies of breastfeeding practices in HBsAg-positive mothers have not demonstrated any increased risk of infection to the infants; therefore, the AAP encourages women with HBV to breastfeed their infants. Finally, because a small percentage of infants will not develop a durable response to the vaccine, it is worthwhile to take the joyful occasion of a newborn infant to make sure that all close family members and contacts are adequately vaccinated against the HBV and hepatitis A virus to further decrease the risk to the child.

References

1. Wasley A, Grytdal S, Gallagher K. Surveillance for acute viral hepatitis United States, 2006. *MMWR Surveill Summ.* 2008;57(2):1-24.
2. Lee C, Gong Y, Brok J, Boxall EH, Gluud C. Hepatitis B immunisation for newborn infants of hepatitis B surface antigen-positive mothers. *Cochrane Database Syst Rev.* 2006;(2):CD004790.
3. Centers for Disease Control (CDC). Assessing completeness of perinatal hepatitis B virus infection reporting through comparison of immunization program and surveillance data–United States. *MMWR Morb Mortal Wkly Rep.* 2011;60(13):410-413.
4. Haber BA, Block JM, Jonas MM, et al. Recommendations for screening, monitoring, and referral of pediatric chronic hepatitis B. *Pediatrics.* 2009;124(5):e1007-e1013.
5. Mast EE, Margolis HS, Fiore AE, et al. A comprehensive immunization strategy to eliminate transmission of hepatitis B virus infection in the United States: recommendations of the Advisory Committee on Immunization Practices (ACIP) part 1: immunization of infants, children, and adolescents. *MMWR Recomm Rep.* 2005 Dec;54(RR-16):1-31.
6. Saari TN. Immunization of preterm and low birth weight infants. American Academy of Pediatrics Committee on Infectious Diseases. *Pediatrics.* 2003;112(1 pt 1):193-198.
7. Burk RD, Hwang LY, Ho GY, Shafritz DA, Beasley RP. Outcome of perinatal hepatitis B virus exposure is dependent on maternal virus load. *J Infect Dis.* 1994;170(6):1418-1423.
8. Barlow CF, Priebe CJ, Mulliken JB, et al. Spastic diplegia as a complication of interferon Alfa-2a treatment of hemangiomas of infancy. *J Pediatr.* 1998;132(3 pt 1):527-530.
9. Jonas MM, Block JM, Haber BA, et al. Treatment of children with chronic hepatitis B virus infection in the United States: patient selection and therapeutic options. *Hepatology.* 2010;52(6):2192-2205.

WHAT IS THE CORRECT MANAGEMENT AND FOLLOW-UP FOR INFANTS WHOSE MOTHERS ARE INFECTED WITH HEPATITIS C?

Janis M. Stoll, MD and Maureen M. Jonas, MD

Hepatitis C virus (HCV) is a simple ribonucleic acid (RNA) virus that infects hepatocytes and is an important cause of chronic liver disease in children and adults. Prior to 1992, transfusion of blood products was the leading cause of hepatitis C transmission in the United States. With the ability to screen for HCV in blood products, vertical transmission from mother to child has become the main source of HCV acquisition in the United States pediatric population.

Seroprevalence of hepatitis C antibody among pregnant women in the United States has been estimated at 1% to 2%; however, the proportion of these women that are viremic is not known. The risk of perinatal transmission from infected pregnant women ranges from 2% to 6%. Studies estimate that 10,000 to 60,000 infants are infected with HCV worldwide per year due to vertical transmission. Thus, it is important to know what testing to do for infants born to HCV-infected mothers.

The Centers for Disease Control and Prevention (CDC) recommends that all women at risk for HCV infection be tested at their first prenatal visit. High risk women include those having had blood products or organ transplantation prior to 1992 or with a history of intravenous drug use. As of now, there is no hepatitis C vaccine or other therapy approved by the Food and Drug Administration to administer to an HCV-infected mother or to her newborn during the perinatal period.

Tests for HCV include antibody testing with an enzyme immunoassay test and detection of the virus itself by a polymerase chain reaction (PCR) for HCV RNA. RNA assays are either qualitative or quantitative. We recommend qualitative testing to assess for the presence or absence of viremia, while quantitative testing is used before and during treatment to determine the response to therapy. HCV genotyping is performed on all patients prior to initiating therapy. Although there are currently at least 6 HCV genotypes with multiple subtypes identified, genotype 1 is most common and identified in 60% to 70% of HCV-infected patients in the United States. Genotypes 2 and 3 comprise about one-third of cases and genotypes 4, 5, and 6 are rare in the United States.

Perinatal transmission of HCV occurs only when women are positive for HCV RNA at the time of delivery. Transmission rates of HCV are greater in pregnant women coinfected with the human immunodeficiency virus (HIV) and women who have high viral loads (titers above 10^5 to 10^6 copies/mL). Elective Caesarean delivery has not been shown to decrease transmission

Table 9-1

Interpretation of Hepatitis C Virus Testing Using Age, Hepatitis C Virus Antibody, and Hepatitis C Virus Qualitative Ribonucleic Acid

Age	HCV Antibody	HCV Qualitative RNA	Interpretation
Younger than 18 months	Positive	Not done	Difficult to assess due to maternal antibody transmission
	Positive	Positive	HCV infected, may be transient or persistent
Older than 18 months	Positive	Negative	HCV clearance or false positive
	Positive	Positive	HCV infected

rate. However, Caesarean delivery may have a protective effect in HCV-infected women with HIV coinfection. Fetal scalp monitoring, prolonged rupture of membranes greater than 6 hours, and amniocentesis are not recommended in mothers who are HCV infected. Serum antibodies to HCV and HCV RNA have been detected in colostrum in low levels, but HCV transmission rates are similar between breast- and bottlefed infants. Therefore, breastfeeding has not been contra-indicated for infants born to HCV-infected mothers unless the mother has cracked or bleeding nipples.

Infants born to anti-HCV positive mothers typically have passively acquired maternal HCV-antibody that can persist for up to 18 months. Therefore, we recommend HCV antibody testing not be performed until after 18 months of age. HCV RNA PCR testing is available for infants prior to 18 months if early diagnosis is desired, although the sensitivity of HCV RNA PCR testing increases with age. The sensitivity of HCV RNA testing at birth is 22% and increases to 70% to 85% after 1 month of age that may reflect the variable incubation period of the virus. In addition, some infants who are viremic in the first few years of life clear the infection spontaneously. Infants are considered infected with HCV if they have HCV RNA PCR positivity on 2 separate tests separated by weeks to months. Infants with a positive HCV antibody titer are considered to have had either transient viremia or spontaneous HCV viral clearance if subsequent HCV RNA tests are negative. Table 9-1 and Figure 9-1 outline the interpretation of the testing results and our diagnostic algorithm.

Spontaneous viral clearance can occur in up to 20% to 45% of children infected by vertical transmission. Infants who remain positive for HCV RNA after 3 years of age are unlikely to clear the virus without treatment. Of individuals with chronic HCV, 10% to 20% go on to develop cirrhosis in adulthood and about 20% of those develop hepatocellular carcinoma, but progression to cirrhosis is uncommon during the pediatric years. Factors associated with an increased rate of progression of fibrosis include immunosuppression, obesity, and chronic alcohol ingestion.

The majority of children infected with HCV are asymptomatic but some may have intermit-tently or persistently elevated aspartate aminotransferase/alanine aminotransferase and hepato-megaly. Children older than 3 years with chronic hepatitis C should be followed by experienced specialists who will closely follow the clinical exam and laboratory data and assist families with

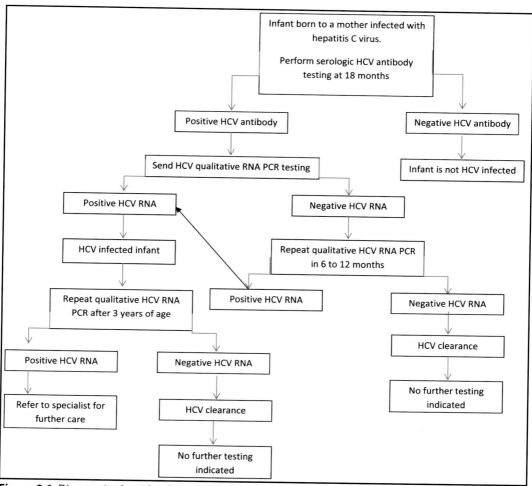

Figure 9-1. Diagnostic algorithm for an infant born to a mother infected with HCV.

treatment decisions. Our decision to start therapy is individualized and multifactorial and includes factors, such as the patient's overall clinical, laboratory, and possibly histopathologic status, the presence of comorbid conditions, as well as patient and parent readiness to begin a strict medication regimen with potential side effects.

All patients with chronic HCV should have the HCV genotype determined to give prognostic information regarding treatment response and need for liver biopsy. The goal of HCV therapy is to achieve sustained virologic response (SVR), defined as undetectable HCV RNA at 6 months following the end of therapy. Successful therapy with current regimens is more likely in patients with HCV genotypes 2 and 3 (76%) than those with genotype 1 (46%).

Liver biopsies can be used in HCV patients to identify the degree of fibrosis in patients being considered for treatment. Children with HCV genotype 2 or 3 typically do not need a liver biopsy as they have a high likelihood of good response to therapy. A liver biopsy may be helpful in patients with HCV genotype 1 who are older than 5 years or those with comorbidities in whom treatment is being contemplated.

FDA-approved therapy for HCV in children is the combination of pegylated interferon (given subcutaneously once a week) with ribavirin (given orally twice a day). These medications are licensed for children as young as 3 years. Children with genotype 2 or 3 are typically treated for 24 weeks.

Children with genotype 1 are treated for 48 weeks, although treatment algorithms are adjusted based upon virologic response. The most common side effects of interferon-alfa include flu-like symptoms, neutropenia, and neuropsychiatric symptoms, including irritability, insomnia, and depression. Ribavirin causes dose-dependent hemolytic anemia and is considered both a teratogen and a mutagen. Contraindications to treatment include pregnancy, underlying autoimmune disorders, and organ transplants, as well as psychosocial factors such as serious psychiatric disorders and patient and/or family unpreparedness. These therapies are generally better tolerated in childhood and adolescence than in adulthood; however, side effects can still interfere with daily activities.

Boceprevir and telaprevir, 2 protease inhibitors, have recently been approved for use in combination with peginterferon and ribavirin to treat genotype 1 HCV infection in adults. Triple therapy has demonstrated improved SVR (70% to 80%) in this group. Clinical trials using these protease inhibitors in pediatric patients have just begun.

Patients with advanced fibrosis and cirrhosis due to HCV should be followed with yearly ultrasounds and serum alpha-fetoprotein measurements as surveillance for hepatocellular carcinoma. The youngest reported cases of this complication were aged 18 years. All children with chronic hepatitis C should be immunized against hepatitis A and B because of the risk of severe hepatitis from these infections in patients with chronic liver disease.

Specific household precautions are recommended to avoid infections from household equipment that may have been contaminated with blood. This includes not sharing razors, nail clippers, toothbrushes, or pierced earrings and exercising caution when managing wounds at home. Universal precautions, as are already recommended for all children, should be used at daycare and school, but patients with HCV should never be excluded from school or activities based on their HCV infection status. The HCV antibody is not a protective antibody and patients who have cleared their HCV RNA can become infected again after an exposure through shared needles. Patients with HCV should be counseled to avoid long-term hepatotoxic medications (appropriate doses of acetaminophen given sporadically are not contraindicated) and alcohol ingestion, and should contact their physicians if they have questions regarding prescription, over-the-counter, or herbal medications that may affect the liver.

Conclusion

Our key recommendations for the diagnosis and management of infants born to a hepatitis C-infected mother include the following:

- Perform serologic antibody testing at 18 months in any infant born to a mother who is HCV positive. HCV RNA PCR testing can be done sooner for families who desire early diagnosis but may not accurately reflect the persistence of infection into childhood.

- Children are considered HCV infected with 2 positive qualitative HCV RNA PCR tests separated by weeks to months.

- Children are eligible for therapy after 3 years of age. Genotype, comorbid conditions, and parent/child readiness are all used to determine if and when to initiate treatment.

- Peginterferon and ribavirin are approved for use in HCV-infected children.

- Bloodborne pathogen household precautions and vaccination for hepatitis A and B should be implemented for all children with HCV.

Bibliography

American Academy of Pediatrics. Hepatitis C. In: Pickering LK, ed. *Red Bood: 2009 Report of the Committee on Infectious Diseases*. 28th ed. Elk Grove Village, IL: American Academy of Pediatrics; 2009:357-360.

Arshad M, El-Kamary SS, Jhaveri K. Hepatitis C virus infection during pregnancy and the newborn period. *J Viral Hepatology*. 2011;18(4):229-236.

Davison SM, Mieli-Vergani G, Sira J, Kelly DA. Perinatal hepatitis C virus infection: diagnosis and management. *Arch Dis Child*. 2006;91:781-785.

Goldberg E, Chopra S, O'Donovan DJ. Perinatal transmission of hepatitis C cirus. *UpToDate* 2001;ed 19.3. www.uptodateonline.com. Accessed January 1, 2012.

Jonas MM. Hepatitis C virus infection in children. *UpToDate* 2011;ed 19.3. www.uptodateonline.com. Accessed January 1, 2012.

Yeung LTF, King SM, Roberts EA. Mother-to-infant transmission of hepatitis C virus. *Hepatology*. 2001;34(2):223-229.

SECTION II

PATIENTS WITH
STATIC ENCEPHALOPATHY

10

How Do I Assure Adequate Nutrition Support for the Child or Adolescent With Static Encephalopathy and When Should I Consider Supplemental Enteral Support Such as Gastrostomy Feeding?

Edwin F. Simpser, MD

Providing pediatric care to a child or adolescent with static encephalopathy can be quite challenging given the multiplicity of medical and psychosocial issues. The nutritional care of such a patient often comes to the forefront, in particular because it is such a key aspect of the parents' desire to nurture their severely affected child or adolescent. Indeed parents often focus on the ability to nourish their child or adolescent with a sense that this is the one (and maybe only) area in which they can be an active participant.

Abnormality in nutritional status is extremely common in this population. While there is a subgroup that may become overweight, you are much more likely to diagnose under nutrition in this group of children. Most studies of nutritional status and the effect of malnutrition in neurologically impaired children have been in those with quadriplegic cerebral palsy. Nutritional support in this population has been shown to improve subcutaneous energy stores, muscle mass, impairment of the immune system, and neuromuscular function. Some studies[1] have shown decreased irritability and spasticity, healing of decubitus ulcers, improved peripheral circulation, and general improvement in well being.

Our usual approach to assessing nutritional status is often not completely accurate in children with static encephalopathy. Many of these children have low linear and head circumference growth associated with their severe brain injury. Correlating weight for height and even simply measuring height can be difficult, especially in the child or adolescent with contractures, spasticity, scoliosis, or the inability to stand. My approach is to follow changes in weight closely, utilize knee height measurements for stature, and occasionally use skinfold thickness measurements to assess muscle and fat mass. Unless you have a practice with a significant number of these children it is unlikely that you will have staff trained in measuring and interpreting knee height or skinfold thickness. It is prudent, therefore, to use the services of an experienced and knowledgeable dietitian to assist you in assessing nutritional status of these children. For those without access to such a professional, you could reference an excellent chapter on nutrition in children with cerebral palsy by Bandini et al.[2]

Another important aspect of assessing nutritional status in this population is their vitamin and mineral status. Bone fractures are a significant problem in many children with neurological impairment due to multiple factors. Many of these children are on a variety of anticonvulsant medications, and alterations in vitamin D and calcium metabolism have been shown to occur. Therefore, these children should be monitored carefully to ensure that vitamin D and calcium levels are adequate for healthy bone development. Certain anticonvulsants, valproic acid in particular, have been shown to affect carnitine metabolism. While the impact of this decreased carnitine level is unclear, it seems prudent to measure and supplement if carnitine levels are low.

If you have assessed that a child or adolescent has an abnormality in nutritional status (over or under weight), the next step is to evaluate the etiology of this abnormality to help guide the approach to improvement. For the pediatric patient that is overweight, excess caloric intake over energy requirements is usually the culprit. While screening for endocrine abnormalities should likely be done, we rarely find any treatable cause for obesity. Indeed, those children with low tone, well-controlled seizures, and minimal if any mobility often have extremely low energy requirements. It is essential to try to maintain adequate protein levels while reducing caloric intake in this group. Do not be surprised that you may need to go as low as 30 to 40 calories per kilogram a day to manage the obesity. This can be a challenging task and may require the assistance of a dietitian with specific experience in managing this subgroup of patients.

Under nutrition is certainly a much more common problem in this population. First an evaluation of the adequacy of caloric intake is required. If your assessment is that the child's caloric intake is adequate and yet is still undernourished, I would suggest thinking about two possibilities, high energy needs and loss of calories. In children who have spasticity and frequent seizures, their energy requirements may be higher than an otherwise healthy child or adolescent and indeed their intake is not adequate for them. A trial of increased caloric intake (if possible) is worthwhile in such a patient. Other possible causes for seemingly adequate intake and poor nutritional status may include losses either from malabsorption/maldigestion or from vomiting. The latter is much more likely, at times, caused by a central nervous system abnormality (eg, hydrocephalus) but much more often by gastroesophageal reflux (GER) and/or gastrointestinal dysmotility. One should try to minimize these reflux-related losses by modifying the approach to feeding, such as smaller more frequent feeds or utilize certain formulas that may empty from the stomach more quickly (eg, hydrolysates and formulas lower in long chain fat). In a child or adolescent already on tube feedings, one can try continuous or drip feedings instead of bolus feedings, or consider a gastrojejunal tube to bypass the stomach and avoid reflux or vomiting. Please recognize that jejunal feeds are always given continuously as the small bowel cannot tolerate bolus feeds. We have a limited number of medications with limited efficacy for this problem. Metoclopramide may help some children, although many parents are reluctant to use it because it lowers the seizure threshold. Low-dose erythromycin can sometimes be helpful in improving their gastric emptying, but I have rarely found it sufficient in this particular situation.

Inadequate caloric intake remains by far the most frequent reason for under nutrition in children with static encephalopathy. The primary etiologies are feeding disorders caused by poor oral motor function, poor pharyngeal and swallowing function with the risk of aspiration, as well as severe GER and dysmotility contributing to aversive feeding behaviors.[3] Indeed, studies have shown that feeding sessions with some of these children are exhausting both for the child or adolescent and for the caregiver and often the energy expended by the child during these feeding attempts outstrips the intake. Nonsurgical approaches to this problem include multidisciplinary assessment of swallowing utilizing video fluoroscopy or flexible endoscopic evaluation of swallowing and then treatment with a multidisciplinary team, including occupational and speech therapists, pediatric gastroenterologists, and often even behavioral therapists.[4] At times some simple modifications such as adaptive seating devices to maintain better positioning for feeding or texture modifications can be helpful. Parents may need to be trained in the most efficient and safe way to feed their child or adolescent. As noted, aggressive treatment of symptoms of GER and vomiting utilizing acid suppression and antireflux or motility agents should be tried but are often inadequate.

In many cases our medical approaches to managing under nutrition in children with static encephalopathy fall short. We are then challenged with advising families about surgical approaches. This is a time where we should have a focused discussion with parents about their goals of care for their child or adolescent. Whenever we begin to talk about surgical interventions in this population, we should clearly understand what we expect to accomplish and how that meshes with the parents understanding (and acceptance) of the long-term prognosis. I have always been a strong advocate for ensuring that parents recognize that they are not necessarily obligated to intervene in the natural course of the child's or adolescent's illness. These are certainly moral and ethical decisions that warrant open discussion between the physician, the parents, and others who may be providing the parents with emotional and spiritual support. I often find that this decision point involves a broader contemplation of the goals of care and possibly the initiation of advance directives.

In a pediatric patient with a severe feeding disorder, a gastrostomy tube can be a portal for nutritional rehabilitation along with providing relief of the stress associated with mealtimes and parental anxiety around nourishing their child or adolescent. Oral feedings can be designed only for pleasure and calorie and micronutrient needs can be delivered via the tube in whatever modality works best (ie, bolus, drip, or some combination). In a child or adolescent with more complicated problems, such as severe GER possibly associated with aspiration, the approach needs to be particularly thoughtful. While some physicians will advocate for an antireflux operation such as a fundoplication, one should recognize that this particular population is likely to have increased morbidity associated with the procedure, particularly with issues of retching and gas bloat. There is anecdotal evidence that children who undergo laparoscopic fundoplication do a bit better. Some physicians will opt for the placement of an endoscopic gastrojejunostomy with continuous feeds as an approach to maintaining adequate nutrition, decreasing GER, and avoiding more involved surgical procedures. As the primary care physician for this patient, you should discuss the various options with the pediatric gastroenterologist and pediatric surgeon so that you can advise the family on the pros and cons of the different approaches.

We should also recognize that in the child or adolescent with swallowing difficulty and aspiration, none of the surgical approaches mentioned will treat the aspiration syndrome. While minimizing reflux will help decrease aspiration of the refluxed material, the child or adolescent is still at risk to aspirate any oral intake and indeed is often aspirating his or her own saliva. We must realize that while we may be helping manage the patient's nutritional problems, we may not be improving ongoing pulmonary complications from chronic aspiration. We should keep this in mind as we consider the risks and benefits of surgical intervention.

As noted, this population is clinically challenging. Primary care physicians should avail themselves of the expertise of multiple health care professionals, including dietitians, occupational and speech therapists, pediatric gastroenterologists, and pediatric surgeons as needed. These families require a tremendous amount of support in both managing their children and making decisions. Despite the challenges of day-to-day practice, we must find adequate time to ensure that we are providing optimal patient- and family-centered care for this most vulnerable population.

References

1. Stallings VA, Charney EB, Davies JC, Cronk CE. Nutrition-related growth failure of children with quadriplegic cerebral palsy. *Dev Med Child Neurol.* 1993;35(2):126-138.
2. Bandini L, Ekvall SW, Stallings V. Cerebral palsy. In: Ekvall SW, VK Ekvall. *Pediatric Nutrition in Chronic Diseases and Developmental Disorders.* New York, New York: Oxford University Press; 2005:87-92
3. Sullivan PB, Lambert B, Rose M, Ford-Adams M, Johnson A, Griffiths P. Prevalence and severity of feeding and nutritional problems in children with neurological impairment: Oxford Feeding Study. *Dev Med Child Neurol.* 2000;42(10):674-680.
4. Schwarz SM, Corredor J, Fisher-Medina J, Cohen J, Rabinowitz S. Diagnosis and treatment of feeding disorders in children with developmental disabilities. *Pediatrics.* 2001;108:671-676.

11

WHAT EVALUATION STRATEGIES AND TREATMENT OPTIONS ARE AVAILABLE TO CHILDREN WITH CEREBRAL PALSY WITH CHRONIC CONSTIPATION?

Nader N. Youssef, MD

Cerebral palsy (CP) is a central nervous system disorder of movement, coordination, and posture, reflecting a nonprogressive abnormality or insult to the immature brain. Because of underlying neurological impairment, children with CP have oral motor dysfunction, diminished abdominal tone, and/or associated decrease in gastrointestinal (GI) motility. All these factors may contribute to problems with colonic dysmotility and chronic constipation. These children will often have a low dietary fiber intake that could be responsible for reduced colonic motility with decreased propulsive activity and slow transit of the luminal contents through the colon. It has also been reported[1] that for children with severe brain damage, chronic constipation was related to delayed transit at the level of left colon and rectum.

Physiology of Defecation

There are several motor patterns normally responsible for the movement of feces through the colon. These include the following:

- Phasic contractions mixing luminal contents
- Powerful high-amplitude propagated contractions (HAPCs) that propel stools to the rectum
- Changes in colonic tone after meals

Colonic motility and tone increase after a meal (gastrocolonic response) and may be significantly diminished in children with CP. The HAPCs are the most powerful contractions found in the large bowel. When the rectal wall is distended in response to the arrival of gas and stools, there is a reflex contraction of the rectum with relaxation of the internal anal sphincter pushing fecal material into the anal canal, where it is now in the "firing" position. A voluntary contraction of the abdominal muscles and relaxation of the pelvic floor will be needed later to push the stool into the anal canal to produce a bowel movement. Any disruption of this sequence of motor events or inability to generate enough coordination has the potential to lead to constipation.

Compounding the problems with impaired physiology of defecation is the mobility limitations of these children. Often in wheel chairs or requiring crutches, these children may be unable to sit or squat on the toilet. During defecation, this eliminates the effect of gravity, reduces the contribution from raised intra-abdominal pressure, and decreases the ability to stabilize the rectum.

Presentation

In children with CP, symptoms may often be underappreciated despite the accepted knowledge that it is a common problem in this population. It may be months or years before appropriate treatment is provided. Such delay is a particular problem in children with disabilities either because it is accepted as an inevitable consequence of the neurological impairment or because a higher priority is given to other aspects of medical management, such as treatment of convulsions or postural deformity. Moreover, communication difficulties compound delay as the child with disabilities is often unable to express the discomfort caused by constipation.

Abdominal pain is a frequently encountered symptom of chronic constipation in those children who are able to give an account. Other symptoms may include diminished appetite, delayed gastric emptying due to an impaired gastrocolonic reflex, or overflow fecal soiling due to a fecal impaction.

Serious Consequences

Acute colonic pseudo-obstruction (ACPO), also known as Ogilvie syndrome or acute colonic ileus, is a serious condition that can be easily misdiagnosed and a patient's presentation ascribed from minor conditions, such as functional constipation, to major conditions, such as mechanical bowel obstruction. ACPO is a distention of the colon caused by decreased motility in the absence of mechanical obstruction. It is important for the physician to be familiar with this entity and its management in order to avoid unnecessary morbidity in these cases. Symptoms of ACPO include nausea, vomiting, abdominal pain, constipation, diarrhea, and fever. Patients with ACPO can have severe complications including ischemic bowel and perforation.

Clinical and Diagnostic Evaluation

After obtaining a thorough history and performing a complete physical examination, a set of focused evaluations should be considered in order to exclude disorders that can cause chronic or refractory constipation in children (Table 11-1).

A plain abdominal film can be useful in assessing the degree of fecal retention and the need for disimpaction at baseline prior to initiation of therapy. If the etiology of chronic constipation is unclear, colonic transit time may be performed using easily available swallowed radio-opaque markers that can be administered orally or via feeding tube.[1] Several methods may be used, but the study generally consists of giving the patient capsules with 24 circular, radio-opaque markers. Abdominal radiographs are then obtained on subsequent days. This test may aid in demonstrating the progression of feces through the large intestine.

Table 11-1
Differential Diagnosis Considerations of Chronic Constipation

Muscle Disorders	
Autoimmune	Myotonic Dystrophy Duchenne Muscular Dystrophy Lupus Scleroderma Dermatomyositis Polymyositis Celiac disease (CD)
GI	Autoimmune myositis Hirschsprung's disease (HD) Crohn's disease
Endocrine	Diabetes mellitus Hypoparathyroidism Hypothyroidism
Metabolic	Mitochondrial cytopathies Cystic fibrosis (CF)
Drugs	Diltiazem Nifedipine Valproate acid Narcotics Muscle relaxants

GI: gastrointestinal; CD: celiac disease; HD: Hirschsprung's disease; CF: cystic fibrosis.

Targeted Treatment Is Key

Diagnosis of constipation is not difficult but prognosis is poor with a 40% failure rate in treatment, especially in those with mega-rectum and persistent abnormalities of defecation dynamics. The choice of treatment regime is crucial and depends upon tailoring the treatment regime to the duration and extent of the constipation.

NUTRITIONAL FACTORS

Feeding problems, secondary to oral-motor impairment, are prevalent in children with disabilities and were reported in nearly 90% of patients in a recent study.[2] As a result, such children are frequently fed low-fiber pureed or mashed foods. Even if tube feeding is used to overcome oral-motor dysfunction, the propriety enteral feeds used are, more often than not, those without fiber supplements. This low-dietary fiber intake coupled with a relatively poor fluid intake (often due to fears of choking and aspiration) contribute significantly to the pathogenesis of chronic constipation in children with disabilities.

PHARMACOLOGICAL FACTORS

Polypharmacy is commonly encountered in children with disabilities who often need medications to control abnormal movements or seizures, intractable pain, or to manage bladder dysfunction. Many of these drugs (eg, anticholinergics and opiates) have a negative effect on both small and large bowel transit time. Sodium valproate, phenothiazines, and baclofen are all known to have constipation as a side effect.

MEDICAL INTERVENTION

In recent years, the use of polyethylene glycol for treatment of constipation has become increasingly popular.[3] The product was initially used with an electrolyte-containing solution and more recently as an iso-osmotic solution without electrolytes. Without the electrolytes, it is virtually tasteless with better compliance.

Therapy with a stimulant laxative, such as senna or bisacodyl, may be necessary when the child goes 2 or 3 days without having a bowel movement in order to prevent fecal impaction. Erythromycin has recently been reported as a potential treatment option for those children with colonic dysmotility.[4]

SURGICAL INTERVENTION

Surgical intervention should be considered when all other less invasive options have been fully exhausted; evaluation by a specialist with significant expertise on motility disorders should be consulted.[5] These patients require a careful documentation of GI motor function. Ascertaining the extent of the GI tract with abnormal function through the use of anorectal, colonic, and GI manometry may provide the surgeon with invaluable information. Different procedures (ie, appendicostomy, cecostomy, and sigmoidostomy) aimed at administering antegrade colonic enemas have been used successfully in children with underlying neurological issues and normal children with refractory slow transit or chronic megacolon and normal proximal colonic motility. The traditional appendicostomy, initially described by Malone,[7] involves creating a conduit, usually a reversed appendix, to the cecum that can be used to administer daily colonic irrigations. In those patients who have a dilated distal colon that has been stretched to "the point of no return," a subtotal colectomy with primary anastomosis may be considered. Those with pancolonic abnormalities may benefit from an ileorectal anastomosis. It is imperative that before performing such a procedure that anorectal evaluation be performed to exclude patients with a nonrelaxing anal sphincter. In those cases where a nonrelaxing anal sphincter is appreciated, a work-up for HD would be warranted and if negative, consider botulinum toxin A for internal anal sphincter achalasia.[7]

Conclusion

Adequate treatment of constipation provides relief for the child and can be observed in neurologically impaired children often as an improvement in appetite or behavior. For instance, the improvement in behavior of children with autism following evacuation of retained feces after constipation is frequently encountered in clinical practice. Early recognition of significant constipation in children with disabilities is therefore important and adequate treatment rests upon both a clear understanding of its pathogenesis and the basic principles of management.

References

1. Staiano A, Del Giudice E. Anorectal manometry and colonic transit in children with brain damage. *Pediatrics.* 1994;94:169-173.
2. Sullivan PB, Lambert B, Ford-Adams M, Griffiths P, Johnson A. The prevalence and severity of feeding and nutritional problems in children with neurological impairment: Oxford Feeding Study. *Dev Med Child Neurol.* 2000;42(10):674-680.
3. Loening-Baucke VA. Factors responsible for persistence of childhood constipation. *J Pediatr Gastroenterol Nutr.* 1987;6:915-922.
4. Bellomo-Brandão MA, Collares EF, da-Costa-Pinto EA. Use of erythromycin in the treatment of severely constipated children. *Braz J Med Biol Res.* 2003;36(10):1391-1396.
5. Pensabene L, Youssef NN, Griffiths JM, Di Lorenzo C. Colonic manometry in children with defecatory disorders. role in diagnosis and management. *Am J Gastroenterol.* 2003;98:1052-1057.
6. Malone PS, Ransley PG, Kiely EM. Preliminary report: the antegrade continence enema. *Lancet.* 1990;336:1217–1218
7. Ciamarra P, Nurko S, Barksdale E, Fishman S, Di Lorenzo C. Internal anal sphincter achalasia in children: clinical characteristics and treatment with Clostridium botulinum toxin. *J Pediatr Gastroenterol Nutr.* 2003;37(3):315-319.

12

WHEN IS IT TIME TO CONSIDER ANTIREFLUX SURGERY IN A CHILD OR ADOLESCENT WITH STATIC ENCEPHALOPATHY?

Judith M. Sondheimer, MD

The simple answer is to consider antireflux surgery when symptoms of reflux are uncontrolled despite maximal medical management and are having an unacceptable impact on quality of life. Like most simple answers, this one hides a more complex situation.

For many reasons children with neurodevelopmental handicaps have an increased risk of gastroesophageal reflux disease and its complications. Some of these children have ineffective or infrequent swallowing that delays esophageal acid clearance. Many spend their days supine and recumbent, a position that increases reflux as much as 6-fold. Some have spasticity, dystonia, hyopotonia, slumped posture, chronic cough, or respiratory obstruction—all stressors that increase intra-abdominal pressure or decrease intrathoracic pressure and promote reflux. Some have scoliosis that produces a bony mechanical barrier to gastric emptying. Some have a hyperactive gag that increases vomiting. Esophagitis is common in these children probably because of chronic reflux. Esophagitis produces anemia, pain, stricture, and potentially esophageal malignancy.

Determining that your patient with neurodevelopmental handicaps has pathologic gastro-esophageal reflux is not difficult. If the history is inconclusive, a continuous record of esophageal pH or the newer technique of impedance tells you whether the amount of reflux is out of the normal range. Unfortunately, this test result does not tell the whole story. It does not require a pathologic level of reflux to cause major problems in children with neurodevelopmental handicaps. It is the child's response to reflux that makes it pathologic. For example, a single episode of reflux per day in a child that cannot protect his or her airway may cause a life-threatening problem. In this instance, even nonpathologic reflux must be prevented.

More important than quantifying the amount of reflux is confirming that reflux is the real cause of the patient's complaints. Documenting symptoms while continuously monitoring esophageal reflux with an intraluminal sensor is sometimes helpful to establish causation. A 50% correlation between a frequently recurring symptom, such as cough, spasticity, or pain behavior and reflux during monitoring, is assumed to indicate that reflux is a precipitating cause of the symptoms. Evidence for this assumption is sketchy.

Other tests may be needed to prove or disprove causation and it is definitely worth taking time to do a thorough evaluation. I have found that asking for a home video of the child while symptomatic is a very helpful starting point for discussion with the family and sometimes leads to a dramatic reorganization of thinking about the symptoms. An upper gastrointestinal (GI) series may reveal an anatomic abnormality such as a hiatus hernia that provokes reflux. The GI series may also reveal another diagnosis (eg, gastric atony, esophageal stricture, achalasia, duodenal stenosis, or other gastric outlet obstruction) that can produce symptoms similar to reflux but that requires other specific therapy. Direct observation during meals and sometimes a fluoroscopic examination during swallowing can tell you if a child is aspirating oral contents, refluxed material, both, or neither. Aspiration of oral contents will not improve with an antireflux procedure. Food refusal is often suspected to be a result of the pain with reflux, but studies have never confirmed this common assumption. In fact, food refusal may worsen after a fundoplication.

Other questions that I ask before considering antireflux surgery are designed to assess the role of nonreflux problems that may produce symptoms suggestive of reflux. The following are just a few questions to consider:

- Is there a gallstone, pancreatitis, or constipation?
- Is the child's encephalopathy really static or have there been recent neurologic changes that could account for the symptoms being blamed on reflux?
- What about orthopedic problems like undetected fractures or rickets?
- What about Munchausen syndrome by proxy?
- What about drug toxicities and interactions?

After I am as sure as I can be that the symptoms are a result of reflux, the next questions I ask include the following:

- What will an antireflux procedure do for this child's major symptom?
- Am I sure that it will prevent aspiration pneumonia or other respiratory disease?
- Will it control vomiting and regurgitation?
- Will it prevent reflux that might occur after placement of a feeding gastrostomy?
- Will it cure erosive esophagitis or prevent its long-term complications any better than good acid blockade?
- Will it improve pain behavior, seizures, or spasticity?
- Will it improve food refusal behavior?

If the answer is no, then I consider other ways to approach the problem. If the answer is yes, then I play the devil's advocate and list all the patient's symptoms that will not change after the fundoplication and all of the problems that could get worse during and after fundoplication. I evaluate the results of previous medical therapy and ask whether it has helped and whether it could be optimized in some way. Then, I try to decide whether the potential symptom improvement outweighs the potential postoperative problems.

Fundoplication will not fix all problems. It will not fix food refusal or a hypersensitive gag reflex. A fundoplication will not improve irritability, seizures, spasticity, screaming spells, or pain if the symptoms are not a result of reflux. It will not prevent aspiration of saliva or oral contents during feeding. It will not immediately cure a reactive airway or cure sleep disturbance that is not caused by reflux.

I sometimes admit patients to the hospital while considering fundoplication just to be sure that the family, the surgeon, and I all agree on the symptoms and how bad they are. A short admission is especially helpful when asking, "Should we do a fundoplication at the same time we place a feeding gastrostomy?" While hospitalized, you can estimate the contribution of reflux versus oral motor problems to the child's symptoms. You can use nasogastric tube feedings under observation to see whether they are associated with an increase or decrease in symptoms. You can maximize medical therapy and try out new therapeutic ideas. Maybe the recalcitrant esophagitis will respond to an increased dose or better compliance with proton pump inhibitors therapy. Maybe the nonambulatory older patient who vomits every feeding will improve with careful attention to maintaining body position. There has been some enthusiasm recently for the use of baclofen in handicapped children with intractable vomiting. The hospital would be a safe place to try out this kind of nonconventional therapy.

What Complications Could Occur With Antireflux Surgery?

The postoperative complications associated with fundoplication are well known (bloating, gagging, retching, gassy distension, dumping syndrome, pain, and dysphagia). Also well known is the fact that children with developmental disabilities are at an increased risk for these adverse outcomes and at an increased risk for postoperative morbidity, mortality, and wrap failure. The more severely disabled the patient, the riskier the procedure becomes. In the era of laparoscopic antireflux surgery, the operative morbidity and mortality in handicapped children is decreased, but it is still significant and postoperative symptoms still occur. If you have never seen a child with retching or dumping syndrome after a fundoplication, it is hard to appreciate the devastation it causes to parents and the patient. The postoperative symptoms are usually transient, but it is important to define transient. It is not a matter of days, but may be months before things improve. I have my patients consult with a surgical colleague about the specific type of surgery and his or her experience.

There is no uniform decision algorithm that assures a good surgical outcome of antireflux surgery. Your handicapped patient's best chance of success after surgery is a good, individualized preoperative assessment; a crystal clear idea of what you expect to accomplish by antireflux surgery; and an honest assessment of whether the benefits of reflux prevention outweigh the impact of the symptoms that may remain after surgery and/or the new symptoms that might be caused by surgery.

Bibiliography

Kawahara H, Okuyama H, Kubota A, et al. Can laparoscopic antireflux surgery improve the quality of life in children with neurologic and neuromuscular handicaps? *J Pediatr Surg.* 2004;39:1761-1765.

Luthold SC, Rochat MK, Bähler P. Disagreement between symptom-reflux association analysis parameters in pediatric gastroesophageal reflux disease investigation. *World J Gastroenterol.* 2010;16:2401-2406

Martinez D, Ginn-Pease ME, Caniano DA. Sequelae of antireflux surgery in profoundly disabled children. *J Pediatr Surg.* 1992;27:267-271.

Omari TI, Benninga MA, Sansom L, Butler RN, Dent J, Davidson GP. Effect of baclofen on esophagogastric motility and gastroesophageal reflux in children with gastroesophageal reflux disease: a randomized controlled trial. *J Pediatr.* 2006;149:468-474.

Vandenplas Y, Rudolph CD, Di Lorenzo C, et al. Pediatric gastroesophageal reflux clinical practice guidelines: joint recommendations of the North American Society for Pediatric Gastroenterology, Hepatology, and Nutrition (NASPGHAN) and the European Society for Pediatric Gastroenterology, Hepatology, and Nutrition (ESPGHAN). *J Pediatr Gastroenterol Nutr.* 2009;49(4):498-547.

SECTION III

DISORDERS OF DEFECATION

WHAT IS THE DIFFERENTIAL DIAGNOSIS FOR A CHILD WITH THE SYMPTOM OF CONSTIPATION AND HOW DOES IT VARY BY AGE?

Lusine Ambartsumyan, MD and Samuel Nurko, MD, MPH

Constipation is common in children of all ages with worldwide prevalence of 0.7% to 29.6%. It accounts for 2.5 million physician visits per year and poses a significant financial burden. Constipation negatively impacts the quality of life of children, both in physical and psychological well being.

Constipation is divided into functional and organic in etiology. Most children have functional constipation and a comprehensive history and physical examination in conjunction with symptom-based criteria are sufficient to make the diagnosis.[1,2] The pediatric Rome III criteria, developed in 2006, define functional constipation by the presence of at least 2 symptoms (Table 13-1) once a week occurring over a period of at least 8 weeks in a child with a developmental age of at least 4 years.[3,4]

Even though the vast majority of patients have functional constipation and do not require any testing (Table 13-2), a large amount of resources and time are devoted to exclude organic pathology. The latter accounts for less than 10% of the cases of constipation[3] and includes anatomic, neuroenteric, neurologic, gastrointestinal (GI), toxic, and metabolic disorders (see Table 13-2).[1,2] The work-up needs to be directed according to the clinical suspicion.

An organic etiology should be suspected in infants and older children who are refractory to medical therapy and/or have red flags on clinical and physical examination.[2] The differential diagnosis varies by age; Table 13-2 shows an outline of differential diagnosis of constipation.

Infants

There is a greater likelihood of an organic etiology in neonates and infants presenting with constipation than older children. A careful history and physical examination provides the necessary diagnostic clues.

History of delayed passage of meconium, defined as greater than 48 hours of life, may indicate Hirschsprung's disease (HD).[2] However, it has been reported that up to one-third of patients with HD may have normal stooling in the neonatal period. HD is a congenital motor disorder of the gut characterized by an absence of intrinsic nerves (ganglion cells) in the distal

---

Table 13-1

Rome III Diagnostic Criteria for Functional Constipation

Two or more of the following symptoms at least once per week for at least 2 months prior to diagnosis:

- Two or fewer defecations per week
- At least one episode of fecal incontinence per week
- Stool retentive posturing
- Painful or hard bowel movements
- Large diameter stools that could obstruct the toilet
- Presence of a large fecal mass in the abdomen or rectum

Adapted from Rasquin A, Di Lorenzo C, Forbes D, et al. Childhood functional gastrointestinal disorders: child/adolescent. *Gastroenterology.* 2006;130(5)1527-1537.

Table 13-2

Differential Diagnosis of Functional Constipation and Recommended Evaluation When an Organic Pathology Is Suspected

Differential Diagnosis	Diagnostic Evaluation
Functional Constipation	History and physical examination
	Use Rome III criteria
	No tests necessary
	Plain radiograph of the abdomen lacks sensitivity and specificity
Neuroenteric	
HD	Anorectal manometry (ARM): good screening to exclude HD in children aged >3 months
IAS achalasia	BE—limited sensitivity to exclude HD
	Diagnosis of HD is established by biopsy
	Rectal suction biopsy
	Full thickness surgical rectal biopsy
	Diagnosis of IAS achalasia is established by a non-relaxing IAS on ARM with normal biopsies

(continued)

Table 13-2 (continued)

Differential Diagnosis of Functional Constipation and Recommended Evaluation When an Organic Pathology Is Suspected

Differential Diagnosis	Diagnostic Evaluation
Neuroenteric	
Intestinal pseudo-obstruction	Colonic transit: radio-paque markers, scintigraphy, and smart pill
Colonic myopathy/ neuropathy	Colonic manometry
	Full thickness rectal biopsy, for special staining
Anatomic Malformations of Colon and Rectum	
Imperforate anus	Physical examination
Anal atresia	Referral to pediatric surgeon, echocardiogram, renal ultrasound, and spine films/lumbar-sacral MRI
Anal or colonic stenosis	
Anteriorly placed anus	
Neurologic	
Spinal dysraphism	Physical examination
Spinal cord tumor or trauma	Cremasteric reflex and anal wink
	Look for pilonidal dimple covered by tuft of hair; midline pigmentary abnormalities of lower spine
Neurologic	
Sacral agenesis	Anorectal manometry: may show changes of neuropathy
Tethered cord	MRI of the spine: gold standard for spinal problems
Myotonic/muscular dystrophy	History
Multiple sclerosis	Physical examination
CP	Specific tests
Metabolic	Specific blood tests
Hypothyroidism	Thyroid studies
Panhypopituitarism	
Hyper-/hypocalcemia	Serum calcium
Hypokalemia	Serum potassium

(continued)

Table 13-2 (continued)
Differential Diagnosis of Functional Constipation and Recommended Evaluation When an Organic Pathology Is Suspected

Differential Diagnosis	Diagnostic Evaluation
Metabolic	
Diabetes mellitus	Fasting glucose
Diabetes insipidus	Serum and urine osmolarity
Drugs/Toxins	
Opiates, phenobarbital Diuretics Methylphenidate Anticholinergics Antimotility agents Antacids/sucrafate Antihypertensives Psychotropics Lead toxicity	History Lead levels Toxicology screen
Other Systemic Disorders	
CD	Celiac serology, endoscopy
CF	Sweat test
CMPI	Elimination diet and future double blind oral challenge
Connective tissue disorders	Allergy testing (serum IgE, RAST, skin prick)
Mitochondrial disorders	Specific blood tests or other tests (muscle biopsy)
Botulism	
Psychiatric Disorders	
Anorexia Bulimia Other	History Psychological evaluation
Sexual abuse	History

HD: Hirschsprung's disease; IAS: internal anal sphincter; ARM: anal-rectal manometry; CP: cerebral palsy; MRI: magnetic resonance imaging; CD: celiac disease; CF: cystic fibrosis; CMPI: cow's milk protein intolerance; IgE: immunoglobulin E; RAST: radioallergosorbent testing.

segments of the intestinal tract. The incidence of HD is approximately 1 in 5000 live births with the male to female ratio ranging from 3:1 to 4:1. In approximately 75% to 80% of patients, the diseased segment is limited to the rectum and the sigmoid. In the remainder, the aganglionic segment may extend proximally to involve the whole colon or rarely the small intestine.

Of note, 30% of patients with HD may have associated chromosomal abnormalities such as trisomy 21, congenital anorectal malformations, and syndromes such as Waardenburg syndrome type 4. In the newborn period, neonates may present with abdominal distention and bilious emesis. Complications such as intestinal obstruction and perforation with accompanying sepsis may be the initial presenting symptoms. It is important to remember that a barium enema in the neonatal period may be normal in patients with HD. Those babies with short aganglionic segments may present in infancy with mild constipation, fecal impactions, and acute intestinal obstructions. Enterocolitis may develop in 15% to 50% of patients and remains the main cause of morbidity and mortality reaching 20% to 50%. The diagnosis of HD is based on histologic findings of aganglionosis, hypertrophy of preganglionic cells, and increased acetylcholinesterase staining in the lamina propria of rectal biopsy tissue. The presence of ganglion cells on rectal suction biopsy excludes HD. If the results are equivocal, then a full thickness surgical biopsy is necessary. In those greater than 3 months of age, anorectal manometry may be used to detect the relaxation of the internal anal sphincter (IAS). Failure of relaxation of the IAS is highly suggestive of HD and must be confirmed with rectal biopsies. Once HD is confirmed the treatment is surgical and patients should be referred to an appropriate medical center for treatment and management.[2]

Constipation may also be the initial presenting symptom in neonates and infants with anorectal malformations. Anorectal malformations are a wide spectrum of congenital malformations affecting the anorectum and the genito-urinary systems ranging in severity from imperforate anal membrane to complete caudal regression.[5] The incidence ranges from 1:3300 to 1:5000 live births with greater than 50% of patients having associated anomalies, including VACTERL association. Anorectal malformations can be identified with a careful perianal examination. Special attention should be paid to the placement and radial corrugations of the anus, rectal tone and caliber, and cremasteric and anal reflexes. A neurological evaluation and assessment for spinal anomalies should be performed. If anorectal or spinal malformation is suspected, a prompt diagnostic work-up and surgical referral is warranted to prevent mortality and life-long morbidity.

Delayed passage of meconium or meconium ileus in the context of poor growth and constipation in a neonate or an infant should raise suspicion of cystic fibrosis and confirmed with a sweat test.[2] Other systemic diseases that may present with infantile constipation include congenital hypothyroidism, panhypopituitarism, and botulism toxin ingestion.[2]

Constipation, particularly in association with severe colic and rectal fissures, may be secondary to cow's milk allergy. Perianal manifestations such as perianal erythema, pruritus, fissuring, history of cow's milk protein allergy (CMPA) in infancy, and personal or family history of allergies in the setting of refractory chronic constipation may indicate CMPA-induced constipation.[1] A 2- to 4-week period of milk-free diet is indicated if constipation secondary to CMPA is strongly suspected.

Children and Adolescents

Constipation in children and adolescents is commonly functional in origin. An organic etiology should be suspected in those who are refractory to medical therapy and/or have red flags on clinical and physical examination.[2]

Short segment HD or a lack of IAS relaxation in the setting of normal rectal biopsies, also known as internal sphincter achalasia, may present in this age group with intractable constipation, abdominal distention, vomiting, and history of enterocolitis.[2] Therefore, anorectal manometry should be used in intractable patients to assess for IAS relaxation even in the setting of normal rectal biopsies.

Clinical suspicion of anorectal malformations should be high in children with associated anomalies in the context of chronic refractory constipation. Approximately 13% to 20% of patients with anorectal malformations may present beyond the neonatal period with as high as 25% in the developing countries. Delay in diagnosis significantly impacts the surgical management and functional outcomes resulting in increased morbidity and mortality ranging from 19% to 35% and 4% to 10%, respectively.

Children and adolescents with neuroenteric abnormalities may present with intractable constipation, recurrent intestinal obstructions, abdominal distention, feeding intolerance, and vomiting. Neuroenteric problems, such as colonic myopathy and neuropathy, intestinal neuronal dysplasia, and chronic intestinal pseudo-obstruction, are characterized by abnormalities of the myenteric plexus or the smooth muscle resulting in abnormal motor function of the intestine. Associated neuropathic or myopathic abnormalities of the skeletal system and visceral organs, such as generalized hypotonia and megabladder, may be present. Gastric emptying, colonic transit, and motility studies can be used to depict specific patterns of abnormalities and distinguish between patients with functional constipation and those with neuropathy and myopathy.[1]

Neurological lesions associated with constipation in children and adolescents may include spinal dysraphism, spinal cord lesions, and tethered cord. A thorough neurological evaluation and a magnetic resonance imaging of the spine may be necessary to evaluate the underlying pathology. An exact mechanism of constipation in these disorders has not been elucidated. Abnormalities in IAS and external anal sphincter function, rectal tone, ability to squeeze, colonic transit, and sensation underlie the possible mechanisms of constipation.

Pelvic floor dyssynergia is defined as the inability to relax the pelvic floor when attempting to defecate. It is characterized by inadequate relaxation or abnormal contraction of the pelvic floor muscles during defecation, and in adults it may respond to biofeedback treatment. There is a wide prevalence ranging from 20% to 81% in the literature. However the impact of treating this entity in children is controversial, and all controlled studies of biofeedback in children have shown no benefit.

CMPA should be considered, particularly in the setting of rectal fissures, and a family history of allergy. Systemic diseases, such as hypothyroidism, CD, hyper/hypocalcemia, hypokalemia, and lead toxicity, may be identified with the appropriate laboratory studies.[2] A careful medication history should be elicited, such as opioids, diuretics, anticholinergics, and psychotropics.[2] History of mixed connective tissue disease, amyloidosis, and scleroderma may present with constipation in this age group.

In children and adolescents with new onset constipation, psychiatric disorders, such as depression, anorexia, and bulimia may be likely. Sexual abuse should be suspected in children and adolescents with perianal manifestations of fissuring/tearing in the context of suggestive clinical history.

References

1. Nurko S. What's the value of diagnostic tools in defecation disorders? *J Pediatr Gstroenterol Nutr.* 2005;41(suppl 1):S53-S55.
2. Constipation Guideline Committee of the North American Society for Pediatric Gastroenterology, Hepatology and Nutrition. Evaluation and treatment of constipation in infants and children: recommendations of the North American Society for Pediatric Gastroenterology, Hepatology and Nutrition. *J Pediatr Gstroenterol Nutr.* 2006;43(3):e1-e13.
3. Mugie SM, Di Lorenzo C, Benninga MA. Constipation in childhood. *Nat Rev Gastroentrol Hepatol.* 2011;8(9):502-511.
4. Rasquin A, Di Lorenzo C, Forbes D, et al. Childhood functional gastrointestinal disorders: child/adolescent. *Gastroenterology.* 2006;130(5):1527-1537.
5. Masi P, Miele E, Staiano A. Pediatric anorectal disorders. *Gastroenterol Clin North Am.* 2008;37(3):709-730, x.

14

QUESTION

How Can I Optimize My Treatment of Constipation and Does This Vary by Age?

Warren P. Bishop, MD

When parents tell me their child is constipated, I first need to understand the problem. It may simply be a problem with fussiness and straining during defecation in an infant, but the parents may be concerned about infrequent stools, hard bowel movements, large or painful stools, leakage of stool, or refusal to use the toilet. A formal definition has been created by a group of experts who met in Rome; their Rome III criteria are listed in Table 14-1. You can see that a child who has at least 2 of the symptoms, or any single symptom plus a fecal impaction on examination, can be diagnosed with constipation.

What Causes Constipation?

There is usually a strong behavioral component to constipation. A child who has recently experienced a very hard, large stool becomes afraid to defecate. When he or she voluntarily holds the next bowel movement, the stool gets harder and drier due to continued absorption of fluid and electrolytes by the rectal mucosa. More feces arrive from above, increasing its size. When this large, hard stool is finally passed, the child's unpleasant experience is repeated. Even worse, the accumulation of the stool has stretched the rectum. This large, flaccid rectum is less able to report the arrival of the next bowel movement, which contributes to perpetuation of the stool-holding tendency. A vicious cycle of voluntary stool holding, reduced sensation of the need to defecate, and painful stools results.

Please note carefully that this situation only applies to children with normal anatomy and bowel function—those whose constipation is purely functional. Particularly in infants, one must also consider whether there is a congenital problem with anorectal anatomy or of neuromuscular function that may be the root cause. Organic causes of constipation are listed in Table 14-2. A discussion of these is beyond the scope of this brief chapter, but remember to think of these problems and to do a careful examination of the abdomen, anorectum, perineum, and lower spine in all constipated children, regardless of age. Any newborn infant with constipation must be assumed to have a congenital problem until proven otherwise. A digital rectal examination is essential for all constipated children. You must do this to assess the external appearance, rule out spinal defects, evaluate sphincter tone, and check for rectal dilatation and fecal impaction.

Table 14-1
Rome III Criteria for Functional Constipation

Older Children/Adolescents (> 4 years of age)	Infants/Toddlers (< 4 years of age)
Must include 2 months of 2 or more of the following occurring at least once per week: • Two or fewer stools in the toilet per week • At least one episode of fecal incontinence per week • History of retentive posturing or excessive volitional stool retention • History of painful or hard bowel movements • Presence of a large fecal mass in the rectum • History of large diameter stools that may obstruct toilet	**Must include 1 month of at least 2 of the following:** • Two or fewer defecations per week • At least one episode per week of incontinence after the acquisition of toilet skills • History of excessive stool retention • History of painful or hard bowel movements • Presence of a large fecal mass in the rectum • History of large-diameter stools that may obstruct the toilet

Table 14-2
Organic Causes of Constipation Presenting in Infancy

Anatomic malformations	Imperforate anus Anteriorly displaced anus Anal stenosis Pelvic mass
Neuropathic conditions	Meningomylocele Tethered cord
Intestinal nerve or muscle disorders	Hirschsprung's disease (HD) Gastroschisis

Table 14-3
Commonly Used Laxatives in Children

	Medication	*Usual Dosage*
Osmotic laxatives	Milk of magnesia	1 to 4 mL/kg/day
	Polyethylene glycol 3350	0.4 to 0.8 g/kg/day
	Lactulose 70% solution	1 to 3 mL/kg/day
	Sorbitol 70% solution	1 to 3 mL/kg/day
Lubricant laxatives	Mineral oil	1 to 4 mL/kg/day
Stimulant laxatives	Bisacodyl	5 to 15 mg/day; avoid continuous use

How Do I Treat Constipation in Children?

Proper treatment of constipation depends upon understanding the cause and doing what is necessary to interrupt it. In the absence of an organic etiology, I have always found that it is important to emphasize that "the real treatment for constipation is using the toilet." Unless toilet sitting is enabled and encouraged, medication alone is seldom sufficient. It is critically important to explain this to both the parents and the child. Of course, what one tells the child must depend upon age and developmental status. Infants are obviously unresponsive to explanations; older children must be encouraged to work on bowel habits. Toilet sitting must be done when there is some chance of success (immediately after meals and upon awakening in the morning). Toddlers must simply be placed on the toilet at these times. All children need to hear a version of why they must do this, as described earlier in, "What causes constipation?" Use of age-appropriate explanations and incentives for making an effort on the potty should be used in all cases. Simple praise, hugs, and parental approval are usually sufficient, but sticker charts or other formal behavioral modification protocols are appropriate in some cases.

Medications for daily use should be nonhabit forming and safe. Osmotic agents increase fecal water content, take away the pain, and make it easier to defecate; these are the mainstay of therapy. Milk of magnesia (MOM) and polyethylene glycol 3350 (PEG) are most commonly used. Nonabsorbable disaccharides like lactulose and sorbitol also increase fecal water content, but often cause gas and cramping because they are fermentable. One may also consider mineral oil, dietary fiber supplements, and stimulants such as bisacodyl and senna. Whatever agent is chosen must be tolerated by the child and used at a dose that softens the stool and increases the frequency of defecation to at least daily. Typical doses of commonly used laxatives are listed in Table 14-3.

If a fecal impaction is present, enemas may be considered, but because these are uncomfortable and unpleasant, I prefer to avoid these as much as possible. I like to use 4 to 5 days of higher-dose oral PEG (1.5 g/kg/day) before reducing the dose to the maintenance doses (see Table 14-3). This is very effective at removing the impaction gently and safely. Repeat rectal examination at the completion of the disimpaction regimen is recommended to assure that the treatment has been effective.

Does Treatment Vary by Age?

The principles of treatment are the same for all ages. First rule out organic causes, then work on bowel habits and, at the same time, assure that stools are soft and easy to pass. With respect to medications, MOM is easiest to use in infants. It is effective, safe, does not require mixing, and is administered in small volumes. However, older children tend to object to its chalky taste, and PEG is, therefore, the treatment of choice in any child old enough to drink it from a cup. PEG was initially marketed in the United States as Miralax; this agent is now available throughout the United States as a generic product as well. It is an inert, minimally absorbed, nontoxic osmotic agent that has the additional desirable property of being nearly tasteless. One capful (17 g) is dissolved in 8 fluid ounces (240 mL) of a clear beverage and is stirred until dissolved. You must instruct parents on how to mix it and how many ounces they must give to deliver the desired dose. I prefer to dissolve the PEG in a sugar-free beverage and to administer it in 2 divided doses. The amount of solution given may be adjusted up or down, in order to achieve adequate softening of stools.

Fiber supplements are seldom adequate to treat constipation by themselves but can be used in addition to an osmotic agent. These can add soft bulk to stools. I avoid mineral oil because of its tendency to leak from the anus and because of theoretical concerns of lipid aspiration and fat-soluble vitamin depletion. I personally avoid nonabsorbable disaccharides like lactulose because they are fermented by colonic bacteria and can cause excessive gas and cramping. Regardless of the choice of laxative, the right dose of laxative for all ages is the dose that works. There is considerable individual variation from child to child, so I encourage families to adjust the dose gradually until soft, comfortable stools are achieved. This will enable the most important aspect of treatment (using the toilet) to proceed with minimal interference from fear and pain.

Bibliography

Constipation Guideline Committee of the North American Society for Pediatric Gastroenterology, Hepatology and Nutrition. Evaluation and treatment of constipation in infants and children: recommendations of the North American Society for Pediatric Gastroenterology, Hepatology and Nutrition. *J Pediatr Gastroenterol Nutr.* 2006;43(3):e1-e13.

Hyman PE, Milla PJ, Benninga MA, Davidson GP, Fleisher DF, Taminiau J. Childhood functional gastrointestinal disorders: neonate/toddler. *Gastroenterology.* 2006;130(5):1519-1526.

North American Society for Pediatric Gastroenterology, Hepatology and Nutrition. Evaluation and treatment of constipation in children: summary of updated recommendations of the North American Society for Pediatric Gastroenterology, Hepatology and Nutrition. *J Pediatr Gastroenterol Nutr.* 2006;43(3):405-407.

Pashankar DS, Bishop WP. Efficacy and optimal dose of daily polyethylene glycol 3350 for treatment of constipation and encopresis in children. *J Pediatr.* 2001;139(3):428-432.

Rasquin A, Di Lorenzo C, Forbes D, et al. Childhood functional gastrointestinal disorders: child/adolescent. *Gastroenterology.* 2006;130(5):1527-1537.

15

WHY DO CHILDREN DEVELOP FECAL INCONTINENCE AND WHAT DIAGNOSTIC EVALUATION AND TREATMENTS ARE BEST FOR THOSE AFFECTED WITH IT?

Vera Loening-Baucke, MD and Alexander Swidsinski, MD

Only 25% to 30% of normal children in the United States are reliably toilet trained by 2 years of age, 80% by 3 years, and 97% by 4 years. The relatively wide range in age for achieving bowel control among normal children influences the definition of fecal incontinence to children who are at least 4 years of age.[1] It is reported to affect 2.8% of 4-year-old children, 1.5% of 7- to 8-year-old children, and 1.6% of 10- to 11-year-old children. Boys are more frequently affected than girls.

Reasons for the Development of Fecal Incontinence

In a primary care clinic, the prevalence rate for fecal incontinence ($\geq$ 1 episode/week) for children 4 to 17 years of age was 4.4%.[1] Organic conditions for fecal incontinence, such as Hirschsprung's disease, anal stenosis, anal atresia with perineal fistula or large anal fissures, were rare. Fecal incontinence is almost always functional, defined as incontinence with no evidence of an inflammatory, anatomic, metabolic, or neoplastic process. Functional fecal incontinence was associated with chronic constipation in 95% (constipation-associated fecal incontinence).[1] The functional fecal incontinence was not associated with constipation or underlying disease in 5% of children (functional nonretentive fecal incontinence).[1]

The etiology of constipation and/or fecal incontinence is mostly unknown and currently assumed to arise from interactions between the central and enteric nervous systems affected by multiple determinants, including genetic predisposition, environmental factors, life stress, psychological state, coping, and social support.

Table 15-1
Clinical Features of Constipation-Associated Fecal Incontinence

History
• Difficulties with defecation began early in life (50% ≤ 1 year of age)
• Passage of enormous stools
• Obstruction of the toilet by stool
• Symptoms due to the increasing accumulation of stool
○ Retentive posturing
○ Abdominal pain and irritability
○ Anal or rectal pain
○ Anorexia
○ Urinary symptoms: urinary incontinence and urinary tract infection
• Unusual behaviors in coping with the fecal incontinence
○ Nonchalant attitude regarding the fecal incontinence
○ Hiding of dirty underwear
○ Lack of awareness of an incontinence episode
• Dramatic disappearance of most symptoms following the passage of a huge stool
Physical and Rectal Examination
• Fecal material on perineum
• Rectum filled with large amount of stool
• Palpable abdominal fecal mass

CONSTIPATION-ASSOCIATED FECAL INCONTINENCE

The features of constipation-associated fecal incontinence are found in Table 15-1. Often the onset of constipation occurs when a child begins toilet training. Another common time is the start of school, when toilet use is regulated to special times and toilets may not be clean and private. Some constipated children will have intermittent fecal incontinence. A period free of fecal incontinence may occur after a huge bowel movement that may obstruct the toilet and fecal incontinence will resume only after several days of stool retention. Usually, the consistency of stool found in the underwear is loose or clay-like. Sometimes the core of the impaction breaks off and is found as a firm stool in the underwear. Stool retention results when stool expulsion has not occurred for many days. The rectum can become so large that the stored stool can be felt as an abdominal mass that sometimes reaches up to the umbilicus or higher. The progressive fecal accumulation in the rectum eventually leads to pelvic floor muscle fatigue, leading to leakage of formed, soft or semi-liquid stools.

FUNCTIONAL NONRETENTIVE FECAL INCONTINENCE

You should recognize that not all children with fecal incontinence have constipation. For these children, approximately 5% of the incontinent children, the term *functional nonretentive fecal incontinence* is used.[2] The diagnostic criteria suggested by the Rome III criteria team[3] for functional nonretentive fecal incontinence are ≥ 1 episode/week for the preceding 2 months in a child of a developmental age (≥ 4 years); a history of defecation into places inappropriate to the social context; and no evidence of an inflammatory, anatomic, metabolic, or neoplastic process considered likely to be an explanation for the subject's symptoms.

Most children with nonretentive fecal incontinence have daily bowel movements and many have complete stool evacuations of normal consistency in their undergarments. The diagnosis is supported by a history of normal frequency of bowel movements and no evidence of constipation by history and physical and rectal examination.

The underlying mechanism for nonretentive fecal incontinence is largely unknown. It has been observed that the frequency of daytime and night-time urinary incontinence is higher compared with constipation-associated fecal incontinence, suggesting an overall delay in the achievement of toilet training or the neglect of normal physiological stimuli to use the toilet. It has been suggested that these children have a higher incidence of psychological problems, but abnormal psychological scores improve significantly after treatment, supporting the notion that the fecal incontinence plays an etiologic role in the occurrence and maintenance of behavior problems in these children.

WHAT DIAGNOSTIC EVALUATIONS ARE NECESSARY FOR A CHILD WITH FECAL INCONTINENCE?

You need to review the intervals, amount, diameter, and consistency of bowel movements deposited into the toilet and of stools deposited into the underwear and the findings on rectal examination. Some children may have daily bowel movements or even several per day but evacuate incompletely, as evidenced by periodic passage of very large amounts of stool of varying consistencies. Have the stools ever clogged the toilet? Is there a history of stool withholding or retentive behavior? Is abdominal pain present? Is urinary incontinence present?

You need to do a thorough physical examination in order to rule out an underlying neurological or anatomical disorder. Is weight and height normal for age? Is an abdominal fecal mass palpable? Does the inspection of the perineum show fecal material? You should do a rectal examination. In most cases, a carefully performed rectal examination causes a minimal degree of physical or emotional trauma to the child. The anal size and location is assessed. A low anal pressure suggests either fecal retention with inhibition of the anal pressure or a disease involving the external or internal anal sphincter, or both. Often the rectum is packed with stool, either of hard consistency or, more commonly, the outside of the fecal impaction feels like clay and the core of the fecal retention is rock hard. There may not be rectal fecal impaction present in a child with a recent large bowel movement and in children with nonretentive fecal incontinence.

Best Treatments

A critical point to emphasize is that failure to appreciate the degree of fecal retention can lead to erroneous treatments, further delaying effective treatment including misdirected psychotherapy.

TREATMENT OF CONSTIPATION-ASSOCIATED FECAL INCONTINENCE

You need to spend time with the child and parents for effective education. You must explain that the bowel movements are perceived as difficult and painful. The child, therefore, associates bowel movements with pain, which leads to stool withholding, which leads to rock-hard stools. Thus, a vicious cycle is started that leads to chronic fecal retention and eventually to fecal incontinence. You need to stress that the fecal incontinence is not caused by a disturbance in the psychological behavior of the child and is not the parents' fault. It occurs usually without the knowledge of the child, although the child may be able to prevent the incontinence for short periods of time if the child concentrates carefully on closing the external anal sphincter and uses the toilet frequently.

If stool retention is present, then you need to disimpact the rectum. You can do this without the use of enemas comfortably at home with oral laxatives, such as polyethylene glycol with or without electrolytes at a dose of 1.5 g/kg bodyweight/day, or milk of magnesia (MOM), mineral oil, or lactulose at a dose of 2 to 3 mL/kg bodyweight/day in usually 3 to 5 days. Oral disimpaction may increase the incontinence for a few days. A phosphate enema, 135 mL, used once, can provide quick relief of a fecal impaction. Afterward, you need to start maintenance therapy that may last months to years. It is critically important that the child be conditioned or reconditioned to normal bowel habits and use the toilet regularly. The child is encouraged to sit on the toilet for up to 5 minutes, 3 to 4 times a day following meals. You should ask the child and parent to keep a daily record of bowel movements, fecal and urinary incontinence, and medication use. This helps to monitor compliance and assists in making appropriate adjustments in the treatment program. If necessary, positive reinforcement and rewards for compliant behavior are given for effort and later for success, using star charts, little presents, television viewing, or computer game time as rewards.

Daily defecation is maintained by the daily administration of laxatives, beginning in the evening of the clinic visit. The most commonly used and preferred laxative by physician and children is polyethylene glycol in a dose of 0.5 to 0.7 g/kg bodyweight/day. Polyethylene glycol is tasteless, odorless, colorless, and has no grit when stirred in juice, flavored beverages, or water for several minutes. Lactulose, sorbitol, or MOM at a dose of 1 to 3 mL/kg bodyweight/day can also be used. The laxative dose depends on bodyweight and severity of the constipation.

TREATMENT OF NONRETENTIVE FECAL INCONTINENCE

The treatment of children with nonretentive fecal incontinence has not been well defined. You should provide education, instructions to fill out a bowel diary, and request strict toilet training (3 times daily, 5 minutes after meals without any distractions). An appropriate diagnosis of functional nonretentive fecal incontinence is significant because these children do not benefit from laxatives.[2,4] You should discuss an additional reward system, such as praise, small gifts, or story or TV time, to enhance motivation.

FOLLOW-UP VISITS AND WEANING FROM MEDICATION

Since the management of fecal incontinence requires considerable patience and effort on the part of the child and parents, you should provide necessary support and encouragement during regularly scheduled office visits. You should assess the progress by reviewing the stool records and repeating the abdominal and, if necessary, the rectal examination. If necessary, adjust the laxative dose. After regular bowel habits are established, the frequency of toilet sitting is reduced and the medication dose is gradually decreased while maintaining one bowel movement daily without fecal incontinence. Once the child feels the urge to defecate and initiates toilet use on his or her own, the scheduled toilet times can be discontinued. After 6 to 12 months, tapering to discontinuation of the medication is attempted. Treatment (laxatives and/or toilet sitting) needs to resume if fecal incontinence recurs.

OUTCOME

Approximately 50% of children with constipation-associated fecal incontinence remain recovered 1 year later, while recovery rates between 48% to 69% were reported at 4 to 10 year follow-up. Although the 2-year recovery rate in children with functional nonretentive fecal incontinence can be as low as 29%, the long-term recovery rates are similar to those with constipation-associated fecal incontinence.

References

1. Loening-Baucke V. Prevalence rates for constipation, fecal incontinence and urinary incontinence in children evaluated in primary care clinics. *Arch Dis Child*. 2006;92:486-489.
2. van Ginkel R, Benninga MA, Blommaart PJE, et al. Lack of benefit of laxatives as adjunctive therapy for functional nonretentive fecal soiling in children. *J Pediatr*. 2000;137:808-813.
3. Rasquin A, Di Lorenzo C, Forbes D, et al. Childhood functional gastrointestinal disorders: child/adolescent. *Gastroenterology*. 2006;130(5):1527-1537.
4. Loening-Baucke V, Swidsinski A. Constipation and fecal incontinence. In: Wyllie R, Hyams JS, Kay M, eds. *Pediatric Gastrointestinal and Liver Disease*. 3rd ed. Philadelphia, PA: Elseiver. 2011:127-135.

SECTION IV

NUTRITION

16

HOW CAN I EFFECTIVELY INTERVENE IN A CHILD THAT IS OVERWEIGHT OR OBESE?

Jeannie Huang, MD, MPH

Intervention in the child that is overweight or obese can appear to be a daunting task to undertake in the clinical office. Many clinicians feel that effective intervention will take too much time and effort. In truth, while it can take time and effort to reduce weight to the normal range in youth, time spent counseling can be reasonable if distributed across visits. In fact, this approach is probably more realistic as the issue demands multiple discussions over time. One has to remember that it took months and even years to achieve the unhealthy weight in the first place. Expecting a "magic pill" surgery or one time discussion to cure the issue is frankly unrealistic.

In general, delivering consistent messages over time works best with families. It is thus important to know the messages that you wish to convey and standardize them. Discuss weight in the context of health from the very beginning. Families are often surprised by the number of diseases associated with obesity and by the fact that many of these conditions (particularly hypertension, type 2 diabetes, and fatty liver disease) often have no symptoms, and yet are associated with significant morbidity and health costs in the future. In regards to behavioral intervention messages, there are existing obesity patient education programs such as 5-2-1-0 (5 fruits and vegetables per day, limit screen time to 2 hours daily, 1 hour of daily physical activity, and 0 [no] sugar-sweetened beverages) and the HOPE (Health and Obesity; Prevention and Education) Project's SHAPES (S, no soda or sugar-sweetened beverages; H, eat at home; A, 1 hour of physical activity daily; P, watch portion sizes; E, eat breakfast daily; and S, no more than 2 hours of screen time daily [Figure 16-1]), with available patient materials that you may purchase or freely download for use in your practice (request at hopeproject@ucsd.edu). By reviewing consistent messages repeatedly, families begin to understand that weight is an important health outcome that deserves monitoring and mention.

One important aspect of intervention is screening for comorbidities. In particular, several comorbidities are asymptomatic until severe disease exists. These include hypertension, type 2 diabetes, and fatty liver disease. Given the lack of symptoms, it is important to screen for these disorders as recommended. Ordering of screening labs based on weight status can often facilitate the discussion regarding health risks and prompt further discussions on what families can do to help prevent future health issues. Once comorbidities are discovered, effective treatment and referral to relevant subspecialists may then be performed for further management. Regardless of

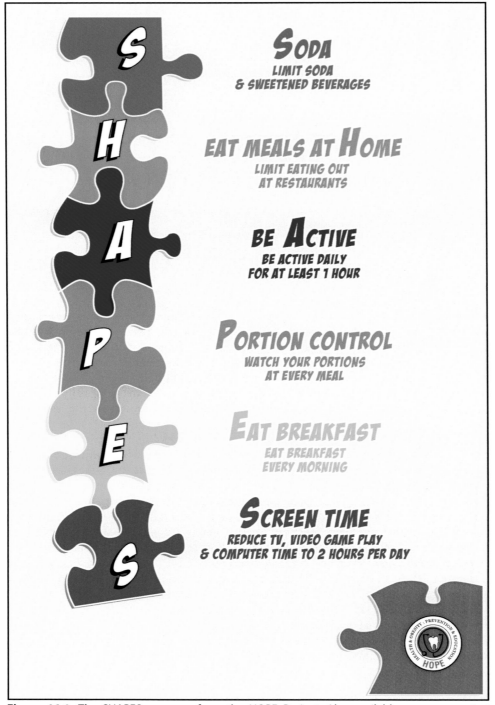

Figure 16-1. The SHAPES message from the HOPE Project. Also available upon request at hopeproject@ucsd.edu.

whether comorbidities are present, it is important to review behavioral intervention messages as a means of prevention. In cases where comorbidities are present, weight management still remains a key factor in treatment and should be presented as such.

In behavioral counseling and weight management, it is important to remember that there are 5 stages to behavioral change, including precontemplation, contemplation, preparation, action, and maintenance and relapse prevention. Recognizing where your patient is in the process of change can allow you to select appropriate and effective counseling messages.

During precontemplation, patients are not thinking about changing their behavior and often are in denial regarding or downplaying the risks associated with their unhealthy behaviors. This can be a challenging phase for counseling; motivational interviewing techniques are most effective. Motivational interviewing incorporates empathy and reflective listening and centers discussions around the patient to effect change.

During contemplation, patients are ambivalent about changing their behavior. It is a time where review of the pros and cons to behavior change should be performed during counseling (this can be done via a handout as well).

During preparation, patients prepare to make a behavioral change. This is an experimental phase and early successes often improve compliance. It is important during this phase to ensure patients make short, achievable, and realistic goals to ensure success.

During the action phase, patients are actively engaging in the desired behavioral change. This is a period of success and patients should be praised to encourage continued performance of desired behaviors.

Maintenance and relapse prevention is next and is often the most difficult phase. Occasional relapses are to be expected and should be prepared for with encouragement and supportive counseling. Goals should be realigned with quick success in mind to encourage resumption of desired behaviors.

When discussing weight, it is important to know to whom you should target the discussion/counseling. Weight management interventions in the pediatric setting must target the parent if the child is immature and/or activities are reliant on the parent. In this scenario, parents are the active agents of change and must support behavioral change via provision of physical activity and dietary resources to ensure success. Research studies demonstrate the crucial role parents play in weight management. If the child is teenaged and no longer reliant on his or her parent for interactions with the environment, it is appropriate to target the adolescent. Regardless, parents will still need to be part of the discussion in adolescent weight management as environmental resources still often remain in the parents' domain while the "child" is living in the parental home.

Sometimes, personalized weight counseling at the physician-patient level is ineffective. It is important to recognize that weight management for refractory cases often requires a team effort. For this reason, many obesity centers have adopted a multidisciplinary approach to weight management. A team approach with representatives from nutrition, physical activity, behavioral change, and social work is frequently needed to have appreciable effects on behavior in families with severe obesity. It would be wise to become familiar with the obesity resources available in your community so that you can access needed referrals when required.

Lastly, as physicians, we are called upon by the Institute of Medicine to not only be active in weight management and engage in the prevention of childhood obesity, but also to act as advocates for our patients in the community. Research has shown that obesity is related to environmental factors in the community, such as access to fruits and vegetables and to places for safe play and physical activity (walkability). Physicians have been and continue to be effective messengers and authorities on obesity prevention issues, and can be instrumental in achieving needed environmental change and public policy to address obesity in their community.

Bibliography

Barlow SE. Expert committee recommendations regarding the prevention, assessment, and treatment of child and adolescent overweight and obesity: summary report. *Pediatrics*. 2007;120 (suppl 4):S164-S192.

Huang J, Pokala P, Hill L, et al. The Health and Obesity: Prevention and Education (HOPE) Curriculum Project–curriculum development. *Pediatrics*. 2009;124(5):1438-1446.

Norcross JC, Krebs PM, Prochaska JO. Stages of change. *J Clin Psychol*. 2011;67(2):143-154.

Schwartz RP. Motivational interviewing (patient-centered counseling) to address childhood obesity. *Pediatr Ann*. 2010;39(3):154-158.

QUESTION 17

WHAT COMORBIDITIES SHOULD I SCREEN FOR IN MY PATIENT WHO IS OBESE?

Nidhi P. Goyal, MD, MPH and Jeffrey B. Schwimmer, MD

Obesity is a national epidemic that has tripled in prevalence in the pediatric population over the last several decades from about 5% in 1980 to 17% in 2004. Thus, as a pediatrician you are likely to encounter obese children on a daily basis. Childhood obesity is associated with comorbidities in multiple organ systems, resulting in significant morbidity, and has the potential to increase the risk of premature death as an adult. It is important to evaluate the obese child in a systematic approach with a history, physical exam, and laboratory evaluation that will allow you to appropriately screen for comorbidities.

History

When approaching an obese child, targeted screening for key symptoms will help uncover specific comorbidities. Begin with a psychosocial assessment to screen for anxiety, depression, and eating disorders. If there are symptoms suggestive of these diagnoses, then prompt referral should be made to a psychologist. Obstructive sleep apnea (OSA) is one of the more common, serious problems that often remains undiagnosed. In order to screen for OSA, questions should include sleep patterns, snoring, daytime fatigue, enuresis, and school performance. A positive screen should lead to evaluation with polysomnography. Type 2 diabetes is an infrequent but serious complication of obesity that often does not have overt symptoms, and thus must be screened for by lab testing. In contrast, 2 other endocrine disorders will have more clues. Girls with polycystic ovarian syndrome (PCOS) may have infrequent menses (less than 9 menses per year) or dysfunctional uterine bleeding. Often, there may also be some degree of hirsutism. Hypothyroidism is an uncommon cause of obesity in the pediatric age group, but you should ask about cold intolerance, fatigue, and other symptoms of hypothyroidism at the initial evaluation.

A thorough review of the musculoskeletal system with questions about hip, knee, and foot complaints is important, as many obese children have orthopedic consequences due to their weight. Back and leg pain are most common and can limit exercise. When pain is present in the hips or knees, one must consider slipped capital femoral epiphysis (SCFE) or Blount disease.

Nonalcoholic fatty liver disease (NAFLD) is now the leading cause of chronic liver disease in both children and adults. Many children will not have overt symptoms, but the most common ones are abdominal pain and fatigue. A challenge is to distinguish right upper quadrant pain due to NAFLD to that caused by gallbladder disease.

Physical Exam

Begin with the vital signs that are crucial in the evaluation of obesity: height, weight, and blood pressure measurement. Body mass index (BMI) should be calculated and plotted at each health visit beginning at the age of 2 years. Obesity in children is defined as a BMI in the ≥95th percentile for age and sex. Around 17 years old in girls there is a crossover with the adult criteria, thus for the older adolescent female a BMI of 30 or greater should be considered as obese regardless of percentile. Obesity uncommonly is a result of underlying endocrine or genetic disorders and height measurement can be a helpful screening tool. A normal height in a pre-pubertal obese patient makes several diagnoses very unlikely, such as hypothyroidism or primary Cushing's syndrome, as they generally lead to pre-pubertal short stature. Conversely any pre-pubertal obese child with short stature and/or developmental delay should be considered as possibly having a genetic syndrome or endocrinopathy. In contrast, short stature is more typical of Prader Willi syndrome in adolescents. Blood pressure measurement is also important for the obese child and it is important to use the proper cuff size, as a small cuff size may falsely over estimate blood pressure. About 13% of overweight children have systolic hypertension and nearly 10% have diastolic hypertension based on age and height percentiles. Three readings of systolic or diastolic measurements >95% for height percentile indicate stage 1 hypertension and require further evaluation.

After obtaining vital signs, you should proceed with a head to toe physical exam focused on key physical findings that warrant additional evaluation in your obese patient. Begin with the general physical exam and take note of the affect and mood of your patient. Could the patient be depressed? The head and neck exam should assess for tonsillar hypertrophy as an evaluation of their airway and possible OSA. Thyromegaly or the presence of a goiter should lead you to further diagnostic testing of thyroid disease. The abdominal exam should focus on liver size as nearly half of patients with biopsy-proven NAFLD have hepatomegaly. Palpating for hepatomegaly can be difficult; however, you can optimize success with a methodical approach. Your patient should be in the supine position with knees flexed to relax the abdominal musculature. Begin with gentle palpation in the right lower quadrant near the anterior superior iliac spine and slowly move up toward the rib cage. Extension below the costal margin is suggestive of hepatomegaly and merits closer evaluation.

A thorough musculoskeletal exam can uncover several comorbidities of obesity that may otherwise be asymptomatic, including Blount disease and SCFE. This should include assessment of gait, passive range of motion, and examination for bowing of the lower extremities. Tibia vara (Blount disease) is characterized by disordered ossification of the proximal tibial physis and is recognized on physical exam with progressive bowing of the lower extremities. Anteroposterior (AP) views of the lower extremities should be obtained in patients with this finding. Evaluation notable for abnormal gait or limited range of motion with passive hip movement should prompt evaluation with bilateral frog-leg views of the hips to rule out SCFE.

Finally, a complete skin exam should be performed. Acanthosis nigricans (AN) is a marker of hyperinsulinemia and has been observed in about 50% of children with biopsy-proven NAFLD. It appears as a hyperpigmentation and velvety thickening of the skin that is usually assessed at the neck but can also be seen in other skin folds such as the axilla. AN can be graded from 0 to 4, based on severity, with zero being no AN visible on the neck. Grade 1 is slight hyperpigmentation visible with close inspection and grade 2 is mild hyperpigmentation on the posterior neck.

Table 17-1
Screening Labs in the Obese Child

Lab	Abnormal Value
AST	>25 U/L
ALT	>25 U/L
Fasting Lipids	
Total cholesterol	≥170 mg/dL
LDL	≥110 mg/dL
Triglycerides	
0 to 9 years	≥75 mg/dL
10 to 19 years	≥90 mg/dL
HDL	≤45 mg/dL
Glucose	
Fasting	≥100 mg/dL

AST: aspartate aminotransferase; ALT: alanine aminotransferase; LDL: low-density lipoprotein; HDL: high-density lipoprotein.

Grade 3 extends to the sternocleidomastoid and grade 4 extends circumferentially around the neck. Additionally, blue striae could be consistent with primary Cushing's syndrome, whereas hirsutism in girls may be a sign of PCOS.

Laboratory Evaluation

According to national guidelines, the following labs should be obtained for all children with a BMI ≥95%: aspartate aminotransferase (AST), alanine aminotransferase (ALT), fasting lipids, and fasting glucose (Table 17-1).

Aspartate Aminotransferase and Alanine Aminotransferase

NAFLD denotes a histological spectrum of disease ranging from steatosis, excess accumulation of triglycerides in the liver, to steatosis with inflammation accompanied by varying degrees of fibrosis. When screening for NAFLD, you should measure serum AST and ALT; however, elevated serum AST and ALT may also unmask other causes of occult liver disease, such as autoimmune hepatitis. Additionally, one must be careful when interpreting normal ranges for AST and ALT as many labs continue to use false ranges for "normal." In a recent study (the liver safety study), it was noted that populations tested for establishing the range for "normal" ALT values likely include children with undiagnosed NAFLD or other liver disease, and the cutoff values are therefore set too high to reliably detect chronic liver disease. The median upper limit of normal for ALT in use at children's hospitals is 53; however, this study demonstrated the 95% levels for ALT in healthy weight and liver disease-free children are 25.8 U/L (boys) and 22.1 U/L (girls). National guidelines suggest that values greater than 2 times the upper limit of normal warrants consultation with a pediatric gastroenterologist. According to the biology-based thresholds, this would be a value of >50 U/L.

FASTING LIPIDS

Lipid abnormalities place patients at risk for atherosclerotic heart disease, and early diagnosis and control of dyslipidemia has been shown to reduce the risk of cardiovascular disease in adulthood. Obese children commonly have a pattern of dyslipidemia with normal to mildly elevated total cholesterol, moderate to severe elevation of serum triglycerides, and low serum high-density lipoprotein (HDL) cholesterol. Mild elevations may be amenable to physical exercise and nutrition with repeat evaluation in 3 to 6 months. More aberrant values, persistent abnormalities despite lifestyle modifications, and mild persistent elevations in patients with a positive family history of cardiovascular disease may require pharmacotherapy.

FASTING INSULIN AND GLUCOSE

National screening guidelines for obese children include a serum fasting glucose and a value ≥126 mg/dL meets diagnostic criteria for diabetes and referral to a pediatric endocrinologist is warranted. Impaired fasting glucose (≥100 mg/dL) indicates an increased risk for developing diabetes as well as associated morbidities such as hypertension. Thus, more intensive medical management is indicated. Fasting insulin is still controversial in use and interpretation in the obese child; however, we find it helpful in our population as it is a relevant biomarker in NAFLD.

ADDITIONAL SCREENING

Table 17-2 lists additional diagnostic evaluations that are relevant for some but not all obese children. Their use should be guided by the patient's history and physical exam. With older age and greater severity of obesity, the likelihood of finding these comorbidities increases even in the absence of overt symptoms. In addition, although not included in guidelines, you are likely to find vitamin D deficiency in many obese children.

Bibliography

Table 17-2
Secondary Guidelines for Comorbidity Testing

History and Physical Exam Findings	Recommended Testing
Hypothyroidism suspected or goiter present	TSH and free T4
Sleep apnea is suspected	Polysomnography
Hip, knee, foot pain, or abnormal musculoskeletal exam	Radiographs of hip, knee, and foot; frog-leg views of hips
Pre-pubertal short stature	Genetics evaluation and thyroid screening
Hirsutism or menstrual irregularities	PCOS evaluation: Plasma 17-OH progesterone, plasma DHEAS, androstenedione, free testosterone, LH, and FSH
Gallbladder disease suspected	RUQ abdominal ultrasound

TSH: thyroid stimulating hormone; T4: thyroxine; PCOS: polycystic ovarian syndrome; LH: luteinizing hormone; FSH: follicle-stimulating hormone; RUQ: right upper quadrant. These should be considered testing rather than screening as they are based upon findings in the history and physical. They also should be performed with the guidance of pediatric subspecialists.

Abrams P, Levitt Katz LE. Metabolic effects of obesity causing disease in childhood. *Curr Opin Endocrinol Diabetes Obes*. 2011;18(1):23-27.

Barlow SE; Expert Committee. Expert committee recommendations regarding the prevention, assessment, and treatment of child and adolescent overweight and obesity: summary report. *Pediatrics*. 2007;120(suppl 4):S164-S192.

Expert Panel on Integrated Guidelines for Cardiovascular Health and Risk Reduction in Children and Adolescents; National Heart, Lung, and Blood Institute. Expert panel on integrated guidelines for cardiovascular health and risk reduction in children and adolescents: summary report. *Pediatrics*. 2011;128(suppl 5):S213-S256

Schwimmer JB, Dunn W, Norman GJ, et al. SAFETY study: alanine aminotransferase cutoff values are set too high for reliable detection of pediatric chronic liver disease. *Gastroenterology*. 2010;138(4):1357-1364.

18

WHAT WORK-UP SHOULD BE CONSIDERED FOR THE INFANT OR TODDLER WHO IS GAINING WEIGHT SLOWLY? WHAT INTERVENTIONS ARE EFFECTIVE?

Frank R. Sinatra, MD

Slow weight gain and/or poor linear growth may be present in up to 10% of infants and toddlers seen in a primary care setting and can occur as a result of multiple medical, environmental, and psychosocial insults. Before considering what type of work-up should be initiated, I try to determine the anthropometric phenotype (Table 18-1). The 3 basic types can be determined by the careful measurement of weight, height, and head circumference. In the first and most common type, weight is most prominently affected while height and head circumference are usually normal. Height may be affected, however, if the infant has suffered from chronic malnutrition. This pattern is usually the result of inadequate intake, absorption, or loss of nutrients or excessive nutrient requirements. In the second type, the weight and height are proportionately decreased and the head circumference is normal. This pattern is most common in infants with endocrine disorders, constitutional growth delay, and primary disorders of bone growth. A decrease in weight, height, and head circumference is seen in the third type and is most often associated with intrauterine growth retardation, metabolic, and central nervous system disorders.

A careful history, physical examination, and determination of the growth failure phenotype should guide the diagnostic evaluation. Screening laboratory studies that have not been suggested from the findings on clinical examination are extremely unlikely to uncover an unsuspected etiology. In the case of an infant with poor weight gain and normal length and head circumference (type 1 phenotype), the first question should be, "Is this infant receiving an adequate diet?" Although a careful dietary history may uncover obvious issues such as problems with breast feeding or inadequate provision or improper preparation of formula, parents often over or underestimate dietary intake. A 3-day dietary record and review by a pediatric dietician will provide a much more accurate assessment of nutrient intake. If it is apparent that an infant is receiving inadequate calories for normal growth, then dietary counseling, initiation of an appropriate diet with adequate calories for catch-up, and careful follow-up may be all that is needed.

If after initiation of such a plan, however, the infant fails to gain weight appropriately, then the questions become, "Is the infant actually getting the prescribed diet? Can the infant take and retain an adequate diet without vomiting, diarrhea, or other gastrointestinal (GI) symptoms? Will the infant grow normally if provided with adequate nutrition?" If there are concerns as to whether

Table 18-1
Phenotype Classes for Infants With Slow Weight Gain and/or Linear Growth

Phenotype	Weight	Height	Head Circumference	Examples of Diagnostic Considerations
Type I	Decreased	Normal	Normal	Inadequate nutrient intake Malabsorption/caloric loss Excessive caloric requirements Psychosocial disorder
Type II	Decreased	Decreased	Normal	Constitutionally delayed growth Genetic short stature Endocrine disorder Primary skeletal disorder Chronic systemic disorder (eg, renal, hepatic)
Type III	Decreased	Decreased	Decreased	Congenital infection Placental dysfunction Genetic/metabolic disorder Neurologic disorder

the infant is actually being given the prescribed diet, it may be necessary to observe the infant in a controlled environment while monitoring caloric intake and weight gain. If GI symptoms are present or develop when the child is placed on an adequate diet, the work-up should then be focused on the primary symptom. For example, in a young infant with persistent emesis and poor weight gain, pyloric stenosis, gastroesophageal reflux disease, intestinal malrotation, and cow milk and/or soy protein allergy may need to be considered. GI imaging may be indicated in this setting. If diarrhea is present, chronic GI or systemic infections, such as giardiasis or human immunodeficiency virus infection, GI allergy, and primary malabsorption disorders may be present. Stool studies for GI pathogens, human immunodeficiency virus (HIV) serology, and a sweat chloride determination for cystic fibrosis would be indicated. Tuberculosis skin testing should be considered in toddlers. If the history suggests that diarrhea began after a specific dietary change, such as the addition of sucrose or gluten into the diet, then primary sucrase-isomaltase deficiency or celiac disease (CD) should be suspected. A low stool pH, abnormal sucrose tolerance test, and resolution of diarrhea after removal of sucrose from the diet would strongly suggest sucrase-isomaltase deficiency. It should be noted that malabsorption may occur in the absence of diarrhea and both cystic fibrosis and CD may present as chronic constipation with abdominal distension and poor weight gain. CD should be highly considered in toddlers receiving gluten-containing diets with both poor weight gain and poor linear growth, with or without GI symptoms, and can be screened for by obtaining serum anti-tissue transglutaminase antibody and total serum IgA (Immunoglobulin A) levels. A positive serum anti-tissue transglutaminase antibody should then be confirmed by a small intestinal biopsy before the diagnosis of CD is made. Constipation, vomiting, abdominal distension, and poor weight gain are also seen in Hirschsprung's disease (HD). Non-GI disorders that should be considered in the type I phenotype group include disorders associated with the both the inability to take adequate calories and/or excessive caloric requirements, such as congenital heart disease and cerebral palsy. Environmental and severe psychosocial factors may also result in poor weight gain despite an apparent adequate diet. A careful psychosocial evaluation and/or observation of weight gain in a controlled setting will usually identify these infants.

In the case of the infant with poor weight gain and linear growth (type II phenotype) chronic systemic disorders, primary growth disorders, endocrine disorders, and chronic malnutrition should be considered. Initial evaluation should include a look at the growth chart to see if the infant is maintaining growth and weight gain parallel to normal or if there is evidence of deceleration in growth velocity and weight gain. A globally small child maintaining his or her own growth curve may indicate constitutionally delayed growth, endocrine dysfunction, or primary skeletal disorder. Measurement of parental height and reviewing the history of parental growth pattern will help indentify constitutionally delayed growth and genetic short stature. A careful physical examination looking for signs of chronic systemic disorders is mandatory and tests for thyroid, renal, and hepatic function should be obtained.

Decreased weight, height, and head circumference (type III phenotype) suggests the possibility of intrauterine growth retardation, genetic or metabolic disorders, and neurologic disorders. Once again, a careful history and physical examination will guide the evaluation. History should include a careful review of potential intrauterine exposure to alcohol, tobacco, and drugs. Birth weight that is low for gestational age may suggest an intrauterine infection or placental dysfunction. A history of recurrent bouts of emesis or lethargy or the presence of hepatosplenomegaly should raise concern about an underlying metabolic disturbance. Initial evaluation should include serology for congenital infections and a careful review of the neonatal screening laboratory studies. The number and types of disorders included in neonatal screens often differ in different states, however, and consultation with a geneticist may be indicated if clinical findings are suggestive.

Although the potential causes of poor weight gain and/or growth in infants and toddlers are innumerable and the potential diagnostic evaluation is exhaustive, it has become clear that the routine use of a large number of studies in a "shotgun" approach is rarely useful or indicated. Admittedly, there may be considerable overlap between the 3 basic phenotypes suggested above, but the classification provides a useful starting point for the initial evaluation. Using the phenotype determined by simple routine measurements and a careful history and physical examination will guide the evaluation in the correct direction in most cases and limit the number of unnecessary diagnostic studies. Definitive diagnosis, in the case of rarer disorders, may require subspecialty consultation.

Bibliography

Baker JP, Dietsky AS, Wesson DE, et al. Nutritional assessment: a comparison of clinical judgment and objective measurements. *N Engl J Med.* 1982;306(16):969-972.

Careaga MG, Kerner JA Jr. A gastroenterologist's approach to failure to thrive [published erratum appears in *Pediatr Ann.* 29(1):742]. *Pediatr Ann.* 2000;29(12):558-567.

Galhagan S, Holmes R. A stepwise approach to evaluation of undernutrition and failure to thrive. *Pediatr Clin North Am.* 1998;45:169-187.

Sills RH. Failure to thrive. The role of clinical and laboratory evaluation. *Am J Dis Child.* 1978;132:967-969.

HOW COMMON IS LACTOSE INTOLERANCE AND HOW CAN I DIAGNOSE IT? IS THERE A DOWNSIDE TO MAKING THE DIAGNOSIS BASED ON HISTORY?

Sonia K. Michail, MD, CPE, FAAP, AGAF

Before addressing these questions, let us first discuss the definition of lactose intolerance. Lactose intolerance refers to the inability, or insufficient ability, to break-down or digest lactose into simple sugars (glucose and galactose) due to decreased levels of the lactase enzyme present in the brush border of the small intestine. Decreased or absent activities of the lactase enzyme in the intestinal mucosa can result in carbohydrate maldigestion. Lactose that is not absorbed by the small bowel is passed rapidly into the colon where it is then converted to short-chain fatty acids and hydrogen gas by the bacterial flora, producing acetate, butyrate, and propionate. Those fatty acids are absorbed by the colonic mucosa, thereby salvaging the malabsorbed lactose for energy utilization. This is a mechanism that patients with low intestinal lactase activity can sometimes adapt to persistent lactose ingestion. Therefore, not all people with lactase deficiency have digestive symptoms, and most individuals can tolerate some amount of lactose in their diet. The production of hydrogen by colonic bacteria serves as the basis for the lactose breath hydrogen test, which is used to diagnose lactose maldigestion.

Lactose intolerance is sometimes confused with the cow's milk-protein allergy. Milk allergy is a reaction of the body's immune system to one or more milk proteins. It is manifested in the first months to years of life, while lactose intolerance occurs more often in adulthood.

But how common is lactose intolerance? There are 3 different types of lactose intolerance: congenital lactose intolerance, primary lactose intolerance, and secondary lactose intolerance. Congenital lactase deficiency is quite rare and manifests itself shortly after birth. Primary lactase deficiency develops over time and usually begins after 5 years of age, when the body begins to become programmed to produce less lactase. Most children with lactase deficiency do not experience gastrointestinal (GI) symptoms until late adolescence or adulthood. Secondary lactase deficiency occurs due to loss of the brush border enzyme, resulting from intestinal diseases such as celiac disease, Crohn's disease, or chemotherapy. This type of lactase deficiency can occur at any age and can affect young individuals, including infants (Table 19-1).

Table 19-1
Types of Lactase Deficiency

Type	Age at Presentation	Prevalence
Congenital lactase deficiency	Shortly after birth	Rare
Primary lactase deficiency	Older children and adults	Most common
Secondary lactase deficiency	Any age	Less common

Primary hypoplactasia is, perhaps, one of the most common GI disorders, affecting approximately 70% of the world's population. Recently, scientists have identified a possible genetic link to primary lactase deficiency that explains the genetic tendency in certain individuals, although the genetic influence can vary from one population to the other. Ethnic and racial populations are differentially afflicted; the condition is least common among Americans of Northern European descent, with a prevalence ranging from 7% to 20%; the incidence rate is 50% among Hispanics; 65% to 75% among Africans and African Americans; 80% to 95% among Native Americans; and exceeds 90% in some populations in eastern Asia.

Infants born prematurely are more likely to have lactase deficiency because the infant's lactase levels do not increase until the third trimester of pregnancy.

How Is Lactose Intolerance Diagnosed?

The diagnosis begins with clinical suspicion based on the history. People with lactose intolerance may feel uncomfortable 30 to 120 minutes after consuming milk or milk products. Symptoms range from mild to severe based on the amount of lactose consumed and the amount a person can tolerate. Common symptoms include the following:

- Abdominal pain
- Gas
- Bloating
- Diarrhea
- Nausea

The diagnosis of lactose intolerance can be difficult to confirm based on symptoms alone. Although individuals may think they suffer from lactose intolerance because they have GI symptoms, other conditions such as irritable bowel syndrome (IBD) can cause similar symptoms. Therefore, the following tests can be used to help confirm its presence (Table 19-2):

- Hydrogen breath test: The patient drinks a lactose-loaded beverage and then the breath is analyzed at regular intervals to measure the amount of hydrogen and methane. Normally, very little hydrogen or methane is detectable in the breath, but undigested lactose produces high levels of these gases. This test is quite reliable with a few exceptions, such as smoking and consumption of some foods and medications prior to the test that may influence the gut bacteria and affect the accuracy of the results.

Table 19-2 **Diagnosing Lactose Intolerance**	
• Clinical presentation	• Disaccharidase assay
• Breath hydrogen testing	• Genetic testing
• Stool pH and reducing substances	

- Stool acidity test: The stool acidity test is used for infants and young children to measure the amount of acid in the stool. Undigested lactose creates lactic acid and other fatty acids that can be detected in a stool sample. This test is the least specific and least sensitive and can be positive in conditions other than lactose intolerance.

- Tissue disaccharidase assay: This is a fairly accurate test that directly assays and quantifies the amount of the lactase enzyme present in the intestinal tissues but the test is not readily available in the primary care setting as it requires endoscopy and tissue biopsy of the small bowel.

- Genetic testing for polymorphisms C/T_{-13910} and G/A_{-22018}.

Is There a Downside to Making the Diagnosis Based on History?

In an otherwise healthy adolescent with typical manifestations of lactose intolerance and no concerning symptoms to suggest an organic etiology, it is reasonable to make a diagnosis based on history and carry out a diagnostic trial of a lactose-free diet, keeping the following in mind:

- Lactose is present in many nondairy products. Therefore, lactose restriction should be comprehensive and inclusive of all foods containing lactose.

- Receiving enough calcium and vitamin D when consuming a lactose-free diet can be challenging and should be addressed when a child is placed on a restricted diet. Also, this is an important reason not to use a lactose-free diet in individuals who are not truly intolerant.

- Closely observe for a complete resolution of symptoms, as partial or no response may indicate the presence of underlying pathology.

If there is partial or lack of improvement with dietary changes, or if the child develops symptoms to suggest an organic etiology that may include fatigue, loss of appetite, GI bleeding, weight loss, or perianal disease, further work-up is recommended not only to confirm or rule out the possibility of lactose intolerance, but also to investigate whether the suspected lactase deficiency is secondary to a disease of the small intestine.

My approach in diagnosing children with suspected lactose intolerance is based on their presentation. If presenting with typical symptoms and in the absence of concerning signs and symptoms, I usually obtain a lactose breath hydrogen test. Since many children with lactose intolerance can have coexisting GI disorders such as functional abdominal pain, if the test returns positive, I trial them on a lactose-restricted diet along with lactase supplementation to see if their symptoms can be solely accounted for on the basis of lactose intolerance. If there is no improvement in their symptoms, I consider other diagnoses. I do not perform endoscopy just to diagnose lactose intolerance, but if the child is undergoing the procedure for a different indication and has symptoms that may suggest lactose intolerance, I usually obtain tissue biopsies for disaccharidase assay. If the biopsies show deficiency, I again trial them on the lactose-restricted diet as discussed with the lactose breath hydrogen test.

Conclusion

- Lactose intolerance is the inability or insufficient ability to digest lactose, a sugar found in milk and milk products.
- Lactose intolerance is caused by a deficiency of the enzyme lactase, which is produced by the cells lining the small intestine.
- Not all people with lactase deficiency have digestive symptoms, and most children with lactose intolerance can tolerate some amount of lactose in their diet.
- People with lactose intolerance may feel uncomfortable after consuming milk and milk products. Symptoms can include abdominal pain, abdominal bloating, gas, diarrhea, and nausea.
- The symptoms of lactose intolerance can be managed with dietary changes but getting enough calcium and vitamin D is a concern for individuals with lactose intolerance when the intake of milk and milk products is restricted. Dietary counseling should be provided to avoid nutritional deficiencies.
- The nutritional challenges of a lactose-free diet preclude its use in individuals who are not truly lactose intolerant.

Acknowledgments

Dr. Michail would like to thank Monica Ramsy for her assistance with this chapter.

Bibliography

Garg M, Gibson PR. Lactose intolerance in inflammatory bowel disease. *Aliment Pharmacol Ther.* 2011;34(9): 1140-1141.

Law D, Conklin J, Pimentel M. Lactose intolerance and the role of the lactose breath test. *Am J Gastroenterol.* 2010;105(8):1726-1728.

Vesa TH, Marteau P, Korpela R. Lactose intolerance. *J Am Coll Nutr.* 2000;19(suppl 2):165S-175S.

QUESTION 20

ARE THERE PATIENT POPULATIONS AT RISK FOR VITAMIN D DEFICIENCY? HOW DO I DIAGNOSE AND TREAT IT?

Francisco A. Sylvester, MD and Ashley Casserino, MD

Vitamin D can be synthesized by humans, and therefore does not meet the conventional definition of a vitamin (vitamins cannot be synthesized by the organism, and therefore need to be provided from exogenous sources). However, adequate vitamin D synthesis depends on sufficient exposure to unfiltered sunlight. Vitamin D synthesis requires exposure to ultraviolet B (UVB) radiation (270 to 300 nm). Cutaneous 7 dehydrocholesterol is photochemically converted by UVB radiation to cholecalciferol. Cholecalciferol then circulates and is hydroxylated in the liver in the 25-position to form calcidiol or 25(OH)D. Subsequently, the kidney hydroxylates calcidiol in the 1-α position to form calcitriol or 1,25(OH)$_2$D, which is the active form of vitamin D.

While vitamin D has been long known for its critical role in the intestinal absorption of calcium, it has more recently been implicated as an important regulator of the immune system. Experimental evidence suggests that vitamin D overall enhances the activity of the innate immune system while dampening the adaptive immune response. These putative roles of vitamin D have sparked much interest in research groups studying cancer and chronic inflammatory diseases, including inflammatory bowel disease. While more research is needed in these areas before specific recommendations can be made regarding supplementation, it is clearly important that health care providers screen their patients at risk for vitamin D deficiency and supplement accordingly to at least preserve adequate calcium absorption and bone mineralization.

Patients may be at risk for vitamin D deficiency for many different reasons. Exposure to UVB radiation is very limited in northern and southern latitudes beyond the 37th parallel during autumn and winter. Heavy air pollution can filter out UVB radiation necessary for vitamin D synthesis. Some patients may not absorb vitamin D due to underlying gastrointestinal (GI), pancreatic, or liver diseases. Increased awareness of the link between sun exposure and skin cancer has prompted individuals to limit unprotected exposure to sunlight and increase the use of sunblock lotions, resulting in decreased vitamin D synthesis in the skin, even in sunny climates. Patients with chronic kidney diseases are also at risk for vitamin D deficiency due to decreased levels of renal 1-α hydroxylase. Certain anticonvulsants (ie, carbamazepine, phenobarbital, and valproic acid) may increase vitamin D catabolism. Individuals with dark skin, homebound, or that remain covered outdoors for religious or other reasons are at risk for deficiency due to the lack of sun exposure. Children with frequent fractures, dark-skinned infants with unexplained irritability, or children with low bone mineral density should be screened for vitamin D deficiency. Lastly, obesity is also a risk factor for deficiency since vitamin D may be sequestered in adipose tissue.

In addition to obtaining a good history of previous and current medical problems in obese individuals, physicians should perform a good diet history to determine which patients are at risk for vitamin D deficiency and need further work-up. Dark-skinned infants that are exclusively breastfed and do not receive a vitamin D supplement are at risk for rickets. Some patients may not consume enough foods that contain vitamin D (oily fish, cod liver oil, shiitake mushrooms, fortified milk, cereal, or bread). A good diet history should ask about vegetarianism/veganism that places patients at risk since many food sources of vitamin D are animal based. A history of vitamin supplement use should also be sought.

At this time, universal screening for vitamin D deficiency is not recommended. However, if a patient is determined to be at risk for vitamin D deficiency according to elements in the history described above, he or she should be screened. The preferred test to evaluate exposure to vitamin D and its stores is 25(OH)D because of its longer half-life and stability compared to $1,25(OH)_2$ D. Based on the concentration of serum 25(OH)D associated with adequate bone mineralization, the Institute of Medicine recently defined vitamin D deficiency as a serum 25(OH)-vitamin D <20 ng/mL.[1] It is possible that extra-skeletal effects of vitamin D may require a higher serum concentration of 25(OH)D than 20 ng/mL, but this has not yet been established.

Children who are vitamin D deficient or have rickets should receive treatment with vitamin D, following guidelines by the American Academy of Pediatrics.[2] Briefly, vitamin D should be given at 1000 IU/day for infants aged <1 month; 1000 to 5000 IU for infants aged 1 to 12 months; and >5000 IU for children aged >12 months. Children with rickets should also receive adequate calcium supplementation (30 to 75 mg/kg/day in 3 divided doses). After healing of rickets or normalization of vitamin D levels, 400 to 1000 IU/day may be sufficient for mainte-nance. Compliance with daily supplementation may be poor, especially in children taking multiple other medications (eg, patients with GI, pancreatic, and liver diseases), so a regimen consisting of 50 000 IU/week for 6 to 8 weeks may be more effective to treat vitamin D deficiency.[3] In children with cholestasis, vitamin D may need to be premixed with water soluble vitamin E (eg, TPGS) to improve its absorption.[4]

Vitamin D supplements are available as vitamin D_3 (cholecalficerol, from animal sources) and vitamin D_2 (ergocalciferol, from plant sources). Vitamin D_3 may be more effective than vitamin D_2 to raise serum 25(OH) levels, but this is controversial.

References

1. Ross AC, Manson JE, Abrams SA, et al. The 2011 report on dietary reference intakes for calcium and vitamin D from the Institute of Medicine: what clinicians need to know. *J Clin Endocrinol Metab.* 2011;96(1):53-58.
2. Misra M, Pacaud D, Petryk A, Collett-Solberg PF, Kappy M. Vitamin D deficiency in children and its management: review of current knowledge and recommendations. *Pediatrics.* 2008;122:398-417.
3. Perrine CG, Sharma AJ, Jefferds ME, Serdula MK, Scanlon KS. Adherence to vitamin D recommendations among US infants. *Pediatrics.* 2010;125:627-632.
4. Argao EA, Heubi JE, Hollis BW, Tsang RC. d-Alpha-tocopheryl polyethylene glycol-1000 succinate enhances the absorption of vitamin D in chronic cholestatic liver disease of infancy and childhood. *Pediatr Res.* 1992;31:146-150.

SECTION V

LIVER

WHAT CONDITIONS COMMONLY CAUSE ELEVATED BILIRUBIN AND AMINOTRANSFERASE LEVELS IN SCHOOL-AGED CHILDREN?

Jaime Echartea, MD and William F. Balistreri, MD

The first consideration in proper interpretation of bilirubin and aminotransferase (alanine aminotransferase [ALT] and aspertate aminotransferase [AST]) levels is to define "abnormal." Despite the widespread use of these tests, the threshold value for detecting liver disease varies with different cutoff values based on the nature of the assay and the age and gender of the patient. Likewise, several different bilirubin assays are currently used to measure total serum bilirubin. The total serum bilirubin is the sum of unconjugated bilirubin, conjugated bilirubin, and a small fraction of conjugated bilirubin that is covalently bound to albumin known as the delta-bilirubin. In the Ektachem Slide Method, the unconjugated bilirubin and conjugated bilirubin levels are measured simultaneously with the use of direct spectrophotometry. On the other hand, the Diazo Method measures the total bilirubin as the sum of direct-reacting bilirubin and indirect bilirubin. Direct bilirubin measurements are calculated as the total sum of conjugated bilirubin and delta bilirubin. The terms *conjugated bilirubin* and *direct bilirubin* should not be used interchangeably. It is important to be familiar with the bilirubin assay used at your institution in order to have an accurate interpretation of abnormal results.

Once you have identified a patient with abnormal liver chemistries, the next step is to differentiate between isolated hyperbilirubinemia versus a clinical picture characterized by a combination of elevated ALT/AST and abnormal bilirubin levels. Any child that presents to your office with jaundice (elevated bilirubin) should undergo fractionation of the bilirubin in order to determine if the problem is unconjugated hyperbilirubinemia versus conjugated hyperbilirubinemia (cholestasis).

The most common conditions that cause unconjugated hyperbilirubinemia in older children are hemolysis (increased production of bilirubin) and Gilbert's syndrome. Conditions that cause hemolysis are hemoglobinopathies and red cell membrane/enzymes defects, including glucose-6-phosphate dehydrogenase deficiency (G6PD) deficiency, spherocytosis, sickle cell disease, and thalassemias, also resulting in unconjugated hyperbilirubinemia. The ethnic background is also important; the frequency of G6PD deficiency is higher in African Americans, Mediterraneans, and Asians. The evaluation for hemolysis includes a complete blood cell count with differential, reticulocyte count, Coombs test, haptoglobin, and lactate dehydrogenase (LDH) levels.

Gilbert's syndrome should be suspected in an otherwise healthy adolescent presenting with fluctuating, mildly elevated levels of unconjugated bilirubin and normal AST/ALT levels. It is frequently suspected on screening chemistries or when mild jaundice is noted during periods of fasting or a viral illness. The genetic basis for this condition is an expansion of thymine-adenine (TA) repeats in the promoter region (TATA box) of the UGT1A1 gene. The end result of these mutations is decreased activity of the enzyme UDP-glucuronosyltransferase and impaired bilirubin glucuronidation. A history of jaundice can often be elicited in other family members. The definitive diagnosis is made by genetic testing screening for UGT1 mutations, but this is rarely done.

Conjugated hyperbilirubinemia (cholestasis) can be caused by either biliary obstruction or hepatocellular disease. Broadly speaking, the most common conditions causing conjugated hyperbilirubinemia in school-aged children can be categorized as biliary tract disorders, infectious, autoimmune, metabolic, and medication induced (Table 21-1).

Causes of biliary obstruction in children include gallbladder disease, choledochal cysts, and primary sclerosing cholangitis (PSC). Gallstones are more common in patients with a history of obesity, hemolytic disease, cystic fibrosis, and Progressive Familial Intrahepatic Cholestasis (PFIC) type 3. Obstruction of the extrahepatic biliary tree can be evaluated with a right, upper quadrant ultrasound looking for cholelithiasis, intrahepatic or bile duct dilation, or biliary sludge. You should obtain serum gamma-glutamyl transferase (GGT), serum bile acid (SBA), and alkaline phosphatase (AP) levels to help establish the presence of a cholestatic process. The GGT and SBA levels are very high in biliary obstruction while the ALT/AST levels are only moderately elevated.

PSC is a chronic hepatobiliary disorder characterized by inflammation of the intrahepatic and/or extrahepatic ducts, leading to narrowing and obliteration of the biliary tree. It presents more commonly in adolescent males with fluctuating jaundice and a history of fatigue, malaise, anorexia, poor growth, and pruritus. Most patients have hepatomegaly at the time of diagnosis. Laboratory clues are elevated ALT/AST levels often with biochemical evidence of cholestasis. Almost all children will have a high GGT level at the time of diagnosis. A definitive diagnosis can be established with a liver biopsy and endoscopic retrograde cholangiopancreatography (ERCP), or magnetic resonance cholangiopancreatography (MRCP) showing the characteristic beaded appearance of the biliary tree. It is important to remember the association of PSC with inflammatory bowel disease (IBD), most commonly ulcerative colitis.

Common causes of hepatocellular injury in older children and adolescents include acute infectious hepatitis, autoimmune hepatitis, Wilson's disease, alpha-1 antitrypsin deficiency, nonalcoholic fatty liver disease (NAFLD), and drug-induced liver injury. Evaluation begins with a thorough history with detailed inquiry into the use of medications (over-the-counter and prescription), herbal preparations, alcohol or drugs in the adolescent patient, a pertinent family history, history of foreign immigration or international adoption, and any history of high-risk behaviors or blood product transfusion. You should search for comorbidities, including obesity, diabetes, insulin resistance, dyslipidemia, or other signs of the metabolic syndrome. Children with a significant (>5-fold) elevation of ALT or AST, with abnormal albumin, bilirubin, or prothrombin time, or with clinical evidence of chronic liver disease and/or hepatic decompensation should undergo an expeditious evaluation.

An elevated level of ALT is more specific for liver pathology because ALT is present in relatively low concentrations in other tissues. Conversely, an isolated elevation of AST should mandate ruling out hemolysis or a myopathic process, since this enzyme is present in high concentrations in red blood cells and muscle. Acute viral disease can cause rhabdomyolysis with a subsequent elevation of AST. Clues for muscle disease are delayed gross motor skills, myalgias, and muscle weakness. The work-up for myopathic process includes obtaining specific muscle enzymes—creatine phosphokinase (CPK), LDH, and aldolase.

Table 21-1

Common Causes of Jaundice and Elevated Aminotransferases in Children and Adolescents

Unconjugated hyperbilirubinemia	Gilbert's syndrome Hemolytic disease • G6PD • Congenital spherocytosis • Sickle cell disease • Thalassemias
Conjugated hyperbilirubinemia caused by obstruction (cholestasis)	Biliary tract disorders • Gallbladder disease (eg, cholelithiasis, choledocholithiasis) • Choledochal cyst • Sclerosing cholangitis
Conjugated hyperbilirubinemia associated with hepatocellular disease	Acute infectious hepatitis • Hepatitis A, B, C • EBV (eg, mononucleosis)
	Autoimmune liver disease • Autoimmune hepatitis type 1 (ANA, ASMA positive) • Autoimmune hepatitis type 2 (Anti-LKM-1 positive)
	Metabolic liver disease • Wilson's disease • Alpha-1 antitrypsin deficiency
	Drug-induced liver injury • Drugs: acetaminophen, amoxicillin-clavulanic acid, sulfonamides, minocycline, erythromycin, OCPs, anabolic steroids, antiepileptics • Toxins: alcohol, herbal preparations, hypervitaminosis A, and synthetic amphetamines
	Other • CD • NAFLD

G6PD: glucose-6-phosphate dehydrogenase deficiency; EBV: Epstein-Barr virus; ANA: antinuclear antibodies; ASMA: anti-smooth muscle antibodies; OCPs: oral contraceptive pills; CD: celiac disease; NAFLD: nonalcoholic fatty liver diseases.

Any child that presents with elevated ALT/AST levels should be screened for acute viral hepatitis, including hepatitis A, B, and C—via assessment of anti-hepatitis A (HAV) IgM/IgG, hepatitis B surgace antigen (HBsAg), anti-HBs, anti-HBc, and anti-hepatitis C (HCV). Hepatitis A infection in adolescents typically presents with nonspecific symptoms of fever, malaise, fatigue, anorexia, nausea, and right upper quandrant (RUQ) abdominal pain, followed by jaundice and dark urine. ALT/AST can be significantly elevated and peak within 1 week of onset of clinical illness. Hepatitis A is a self-limiting disease with no carrier state and, although rare, it can cause fulminant hepatic failure. As such, it is mandatory to obtain a coagulation profile with PT and INR values in order to assess liver synthetic function. Hepatitis B and hepatitis C infections are insidious and commonly asymptomatic in the younger patient. These infections are often discovered while screening liver chemistries for other reasons or in international adoption programs while screening children from foreign countries, where hepatitis B is endemic and most commonly acquired in the perinatal period.

Epstein-Barr virus (EBV) infection should be suspected in any adolescent with a sore throat, pharyngeal exudates, cervical lymphadenopathy, malaise, fatigue, or splenomegaly. The monospot test and EBV serologies are used to assess the status of the disease (previous infection or acute disease). The disease usually resolves spontaneously and affected patients should avoid contact sports until the splenomegaly is resolved.

Autoimmune hepatitis is a progressive inflammatory disease that most commonly presents in adolescent females. Cases have been recognized in patients exposed to certain medications, particularly minocycline. The mode of presentation varies, ranging from acute hepatitis to a more insidious onset characterized by progressive fatigue and relapsing jaundice. A careful physical examination may uncover signs of chronic liver disease (spider angiomata, caput medusa, splenomegaly, ascites, malnutrition, palmar erythema, digital clubbing, or easy bruising). Clues for the diagnosis are elevated ALT/AST, high-IgG levels, and the presence of autoantibodies (anti-nuclear antibody, anti-smooth muscle antibody, anti-liver-kidney-microsomal antibody type 1). You should screen for other associated autoimmune disorders, including CD, in the patient with suspected autoimmune hepatitis (AIH). In 40% of cases, other family members have autoimmune disorders, including IBD, CD, thyroiditis, or diabetes mellitus type I.

An important condition to recognize in the adolescent patient with elevated ALT/AST levels, with or without conjugated hyperbilirubinemia, is Wilson's disease. This is a metabolic liver disorder characterized by impaired copper metabolism, resulting in the accumulation of copper in the liver and subsequently in other organs, including the brain, kidney, and cornea. Wilson's disease is caused by mutations in the ATP7B gene that has a copper transport function, leading to impaired biliary copper excretion. Clinical symptoms are rarely present before 5 years of age and 40% to 60% of patients present in the second decade of life. The hepatic manifestations are highly variable, ranging from asymptomatic elevation of serum ALT/AST levels to fulminant liver disease. Fulminant Wilson's disease can present in adolescents with an acute hepatitis that rapidly progresses to liver failure (ALF) characterized by Coombs-negative hemolytic anemia, extreme jaundice, severe coagulopathy, renal failure, and death if a liver transplant is not performed. Clues are alkaline phosphatase:total bilirubin ratio of <4 and ALT:AST ratio >2.2. In one study, these combined laboratory features had a sensitivity and specificity of 100% in the diagnosis of ALF secondary to Wilson's disease. Kayser-Fleischer (K-F) rings, which are deposits of copper that form a greenish brown ring at the periphery of the cornea, are frequently absent in children who present with hepatic symptoms but without neurologic involvement. A major change in behavior or personality may be the initial presentation in adolescents. The diagnosis of Wilson's disease is suggested by a serum ceruloplasmin level <20 mg/dL, 24-hour urinary copper >40 mcg, and the presence of K-F rings. The diagnosis of Wilson's disease can be established with a liver biopsy for copper quantification; the normal hepatic copper content is <50 mcg/g dry weight and a value >250 mcg/g is consistent with Wilson's disease.

Alpha-1 antitrypsin deficiency is the most common genetic cause of liver disease in children. Alpha-1 antitrypsin is a protease inhibitor derived from the liver that protects tissues from destruction by inhibiting neutrophil proteases. Many different structural variants of alpha-1 antitrypsin exist and these are classified according to the protease inhibitor (Pi) phenotype. PiM alpha-1 antitrypsin is a structural normal variant associated with normal functional activity. On the other hand, homozygous PiZZ alpha-1 antitrypsin deficiency is associated with 85% to 90% reduction in the serum concentration of alpha-1 antitrypsin. The mutant alpha-1 antitrypsin molecules cannot be released into the blood and accumulate in the endoplasmic reticulum of the hepatocyte causing liver disease. Presentation is varied, including neonatal cholestasis, mild elevation of ALT/AST levels in young children, or hepatomegaly with portal hypertension to severe liver dysfunction in late childhood or adolescence. Diagnosis can be established by serum alpha-1 antitrypsin phenotyping.

An important consideration in the evaluation of abnormal liver chemistries is celiac disease. Gluten enteropathy affects 1% of the total population and is a systemic disease rather than a disorder isolated to the gastrointestinal tract. It can present at any age with vague abdominal complaints. However, up to 10% of patients with elevated ALT/AST levels of unclear etiology may have silent celiac disease and need to be screened with a serum tissue transglutaminase level.

Lastly, drug-induced liver injury (DILI) should be an important consideration in your patient with elevated ALT/AST levels. Parents should provide a comprehensive history of medication or herbal use. In children, acetaminophen is a common culprit. Toxic ingestions can cause significant hepatic injury sometimes leading to ALF. The list of medications that can cause abnormal liver chemistries is extensive; however, common offenders that should be sought in the primary care setting are sulfonamides, oral contraceptive pills, erythromycin, steroids, nonsteroidal anti-inflammatory drugs, and antiepileptics (valproate). DILI may present with abnormalities ranging from hepatic disease (increased ALT/AST), purely cholestatic disease, or a mixed picture. It should be suspected in any patient with a history of starting a new drug in the last 3 months, presence of rash or eosinophilia, and cholestasis. It is important to remember that the GGT is a microsomal enzyme that is induced by certain drugs, particularly phenytoin, phenobarbital, and valproic acid.

Bibliography

Bartlett MG, Gourley GR. Assessment of UGT polymorphisms and neonatal jaundice. *Semin Perinatol.* 2011;35(3): 127-33.

Harb R, Thomas DW. Conjugated hyperbilirubinemia: screening and treatment in older infants and children. *Pediatr Rev.* 2007;28(3):83-91.

Korman JD, Volenberg I, Balko J, et al. Pediatric and Adult Acute Liver Failure Study Groups. Screening for Wilson disease in acute liver failure: a comparison of currently available diagnostic tests. *Hepatology.* 2008;48(4): 1167-1174.

Ng V. Laboratory assessment of liver function and injury in children. In: Suchy F, Sokol R, Balistreri W, eds. *Liver Disease in Children.* 3rd ed. New York City, New York: Cambridge University Press; 2007:163-175

Roberts E, Schilsky M. American Association for Study of Liver Diseases (AASLD). Diagnosis and treatment of Wilson disease: an update. *Hepatology.* 2008;47(6):2089-2111.

22

Many of My Obese Patients Have Elevated Liver Chemistries. What Should My Approach Be to This Finding?

Ali A. Mencin, MD and Joel E. Lavine, MD, PhD

As overweight and obesity cases have risen to alarming levels, fatty liver disease has become the most common cause of liver disease and elevated liver enzymes in children.[1] Overweight and obesity cases are now seen at rates of 30% or more in some pediatric populations,[2] and rates of nonalcoholic fatty liver disease (NAFLD) may be 9% in the general pediatric population and up to 17% in older adolescents.[3] NAFLD is a term defined pathologically by the presence of fat deposition in more than 5% of hepatocytes in a clinical context generally associated with insulin resistance. NAFLD can be subdivided into 2 different phenotypes based on the degree of the inflammation and fibrosis seen in the liver. Simple steatosis is a phenotype in which there is fatty infiltration of the liver without any significant inflammation and is generally considered to have a benign course, though there is evidence that adults with this phenotype can sometimes progress to nonalcoholic steatohepatitis (NASH). NASH is the second phenotype, defined pathologically by histologic evidence of inflammation and fibrosis. This latter type is associated with progressive liver disease and can result in cirrhosis. NAFLD can be seen in all populations but has a predilection for males and is found more commonly in Hispanics of Native American ancestry, as well as South Asians and Asians. Despite the fact that NAFLD occurs in a relatively large proportion of obese children, no official screening recommendations are provided yet by academic pediatric societies. Screening strategy is complicated because the disease can only be diagnosed definitively with a liver biopsy and surrogate markers are not yet sufficiently reliable. Serum aminotransfereases, in isolation, do not accurately distinguish between simple steatosis and NASH or predict the severity of disease.

Clinically, NAFLD is generally asymptomatic, though some may complain of right upper quadrant pain as the liver accumulates lipids and the hepatic capsule stretches. An enlarged liver can often be appreciated on physical examination by palpation or percussion. The problem usually is identified at the time of lab testing or when imaging studies are ordered for abdominal complaints. It is worth noting that overweight patients are at risk for a variety of other gastrointestingal related diseases, including reflux, dyspepsia, gallstones, and constipation. Clinicians should be particularly vigilant of NAFLD in patients with signs of the metabolic syndrome that is defined as truncal obesity, insulin resistance, dyslipidemia, and high blood pressure. The metabolic syndrome

Table 22-1
Initial Evaluation for Children With Elevated Liver Enzymes

Assess signs of liver damage	Hepatic function profile GGT
Assess liver function	PT/INR/PTT
Evaluate for metabolic syndrome	Lipid panel Fasting insulin level Fasting glucose Hemoglobin A1C
Diagnostic evaluation	Hepatitis A antibody HBsAg, hepatitis B surface antibody, and hepatitis B core antibody IgG and IgM Hepatitis C antibody Alpha-1 antitrypsin level Ceruloplasm ANA, LKM, ASMA, and anti-soluble liver antigen TSH Ultrasound of the liver, biliary tract, and spleen with doppler study of the hepatic vessels

GGT: gamma-glutamyl transferase; HBsAg: hepatitis B surface antigen; IgG: immunoglobulin G; ANA: antinuclear antibodies; LKM: anti-liver-kidney microsomal antibody; ASMA: anti-smooth muscle antibodies.

has been associated both with the presence of NAFLD as well as disease severity. The lichenified, dark rash of acanthosis nigricans, a sign of insulin resistance, is frequently noted on the back of the neck or other intertrigenous areas of the skin. Alanine aminotransferease (ALT) is often elevated in NAFLD but usually below 150 U/L. Total and direct bilirubin are usually normal. Radiologically, ultrasound demonstrates a "bright" or "echogenic" liver when 30% or more of the liver is infiltrated with fat. Fatty infiltration can also be appreciated on computed tomography or magnetic resonance imaging.

It is important to note that although NAFLD is the most likely cause of elevated liver function tests in pediatrics, it is not the only cause. Other causes of liver disease should be investigated, including screening for viral hepatitis (hepatitis B or C), Wilson's disease, alpha-1 antitrypsin deficiency, and autoimmune hepatitis (Table 22-1). A liver ultrasound should be ordered to exclude biliary tract anomalies, assess for signs of portal hypertension, and evaluate for evidence for fatty infiltration. Baseline liver function should be assessed by ordering coagulation tests. We recommend screening for dyslipidemia and insulin sensitivity since the metabolic syndrome has been strongly correlated with the development and severity of NAFLD. It is rare for a pediatric patient to present with severe liver dysfunction caused by NAFLD, but the clinician should be aware of this possibility. Signs of chronic liver disease such as jaundice, caput medusa, splenomegaly, thrombopenia, spider angiomata, or ascites should prompt a referral to a specialist.

Table 22-2
Initial Management of Suspected Nonalcoholic Fatty Liver Disease

Diet	Three well-balanced meals a day (eg, lean meat, green vegetable, or salad and small portion of rice, bread, or potato)
	High fiber breakfast
	One healthy snack per day (eg, fruit or raw vegetable)
	Avoid fried foods
	Avoid high calorie salad dressings
	Remove fat and skin from meat
	Five to 9 servings of fruits and vegetables per day
	Increase dietary fiber: whole grains, fruits, and vegetables
	Low fat dairy products (skim or 1% milk) to maintain a diet rich in calcium
	Drink 3 to 4 cups of water per day especially with meals
	Eliminate soda and limit juice intake to once per day
	Eliminate unhealthy snacks (eg, candy, potato chips, and ice cream)
	Eliminate fast food
Exercise	Exercise a minimum of 4 to 5 times per week for at least 45 minutes; a vigorous and rapid walk to raise the heart and respiratory rates is sufficient; daily aerobic exercise 1 hour per day is preferred
Other	Limit screen time (eg, television, computer, and mobile devices) to less than 2 hours per day and avoid snacking during this time
	Families should ahdere to the diet and exercise regimen themselves to demonstrate their support and provide a healthy model

In an overweight or obese patient with mildly elevated liver ALT (< 100 U/L), normal coagulation tests, no signs of chronic liver disease, and a negative evaluation for other causes of hepatitis, the most likely etiology of the patient's increased liver enzymes is NAFLD. It is reasonable to advise a diet low in refined sugar and fat as well as recommend moderate to intensive aerobic exercise for 45 minutes at least 5 times per week. Our initial management strategy is outlined in Table 22-2 and is based on the obesity consensus statement published by the American Academy of Pediatrics.[4] It is often helpful to refer patients to a nutritionist to insure compliance with diet and monitor weight loss. The usual dietary culprits include soda, juice, chips, take-out food, excessive high-fat dairy intake, and cooking practices, including frying food and eating fatty meat. Fructose-containing sugars have been associated with NAFLD in clinical studies and animal models, so our group places special emphasis on removing sweets and sugary beverages from the diet. It is encouraged that the entire family adhere to the diet otherwise this intervention is less likely to succeed. Promoting gradual weight loss over 3 months (no more than 6% of body weight total) has been shown to improve NAFLD in adults and it is our experience that maintaining weight in the setting of exercise and improved diet is often enough to improve liver enzyme tests in children. Once a diet and exercise program has been implemented, a liver profile should be repeated in 3 months. If liver enzymes are persistently elevated or worse, we recommend referral to a specialist. If the liver enzymes are improved, repeat testing again in another 2 to 3 months. If liver enzymes normalize, we generally follow patients every 6 months to monitor their weight and repeat liver profiles and coagulation tests yearly thereafter. All patients with persistently elevated liver enzymes that do not normalize or with signs of chronic liver disease should be referred to a specialist to be evaluated for a liver biopsy to definitively diagnose and stage the disease. Liver biopsy remains the gold standard for making the diagnosis and staging liver injury since liver enzymes do not accurately grade hepatic injury. It is important to remember that patients with normal or mildly elevated liver enzymes could have significant inflammation, fibrosis, and even cirrhosis while those with more elevated liver enzymes levels may only have simple steatosis.

For those patients that undergo liver biopsy and are diagnosed with NASH or borderline NASH, there is strong evidence to suggest natural vitamin E given 400 IU twice daily over 96 weeks improves liver injury scores. Vitamin E has been shown to be effective both in adult and pediatric randomized controlled trials comparing post-treatment liver biopsies to baseline.[5,6] Duration of treatment with vitamin E has yet to be determined and potential sequelae from long term vitamin E supplementation has not been evaluated. No recommendations exist for vitamin E in patients who have not undergone liver biopsy or for those with simple steatosis.

Though significant advances have been made in the epidemiology, genetics, and novel imaging techniques as well as treatment of NAFLD, there is still a tremendous amount of work yet to be done. Major priorities for the discipline include determining noninvasive biomarkers for the diagnosis and staging of NAFLD, discovering more effective treatments, and better understanding the long-term natural history of the disease in children. One should consider ordering a liver profile in overweight children, especially in patients with metabolic syndrome. Screening guidelines are being formulated and should be available in the coming year. Early identification of patients is desirable since NASH can be significantly improved with diet, exercise, and vitamin E. If unrecognized until a late stage, NASH can result in significant morbidity, such as liver failure and hepatocellular carcinoma. As the most common chronic liver disease, NAFLD is a major public health challenge. Treatment trials are in progress to find safe and effective therapies for those at risk of progression who fail diet and exercise recommendations.

Bibliography

Barlow SE; Expert Committee. Expert committee recommendations regarding the prevention, assessment, and treatment of child and adolescent overweight and obesity: summary report. *Pediatrics*. 2007;120(suppl 4):S164-S192.

Lavine JE, Schwimmer JB, Van Natta ML, et al. Nonalcoholic Steatohepatitis Clinical Research Network. Effect of vitamin E or metformin for treatment of nonalcoholic fatty liver disease in children and adolescents: the TONIC randomized controlled trial. *JAMA*. 2011;305:1659-1668.

Mencin AA, Lavine JE. Advances in pediatric nonalcoholic fatty liver disease. *Pediatr Clin North Am*. 2011;58: 1375-1392.

Ogden CL, Carroll MD, Curtin LR, Lamb MM, Flegal KM. Prevalence of high body mass index in US children and adolescents, 2007-2008. *JAMA*. 2010;303:242-249.

Sanyal AJ, Chalasani N, Kowdley KV, et al; NASH CRN. Pioglitazone, vitamin E, or placebo for nonalcoholic steatohepatitis. *N Engl J Med*. 2010;362(18):1675-1685.

Schwimmer JB, Deutsch R, Kahen T, Lavine JE, Stanley C, Behling C. Prevalence of fatty liver in children and adolescents. *Pediatrics*. 2006;118:1388-1393.

23

WHAT ROUTINE HEALTH MAINTENANCE SHOULD I ASSURE FOR MY PEDIATRIC PATIENT WHO HAS UNDERGONE LIVER TRANSPLANTATION?

Michael R. Narkewicz, MD

Liver transplantation (LTx) in children is a rare event. Approximately 500 children and adolescents undergo LTx every year in the United States. Since 1989, slightly more than 13,000 liver transplants have been performed in children out of the more than 113,000 LTx performed for all ages (Organ Procurement and Transplantation Network data as of March 9, 2012). Survival has steadily improved and current 5- and 10-year survival rates for pediatric recipients of LTx are consistently over 80%.[1] The age distribution of the recipients of LTx in children is shown in Figure 23-1. Note that 65% of children who receive a LTx are transplanted in the first 5 years of life and 28% in the first year of life. Thus, many children have not been fully immunized prior to their LTx and even if immunized prior to transplantation, they may have had an inadequate immune response. In addition, the effects of chronic immunosuppression on growth, cardiovascular, and renal health are key issues for health maintenance (Table 23-1).

What Are the Key Issues to Consider for Health Maintenance in a Child Who Has Undergone a Liver Transplant?

Health maintenance for children who have undergone LTx should be performed in concert with the child's transplant center, as many centers have specific protocols. The guidelines that follow should be considered in the context of the practices of the center and the unique aspects of the immunosuppression regimen of the specific patient. The mainstay of LTx immunosuppression is calcineurin inhibitor therapy. The 2 most common medications are tacrolimus and cyclosporine. Most centers now use tacrolimus as their primary immunosuppressive medication. Other medications commonly used include corticosteroids and mycophenolic acid with many other options available. The major long-term complications for children include rejection, infection, and post-transplant lymphoproliferative disease.

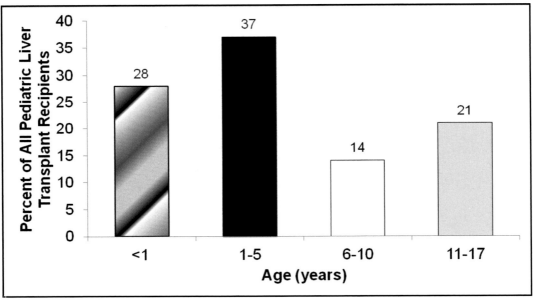

Figure 23-1. Percent distribution of pediatric liver transplant recipients by age.

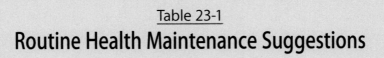

Table 23-1
Routine Health Maintenance Suggestions

- Verify vaccine status and catch up vaccinations as appropriate
- Screen for complications
  - Hypertension
  - Renal dysfunction
  - Hyperlipidemia
  - School performance and learning issues
- Counsel for skin cancer protection

IMMUNIZATIONS

You should review the immunization history of a child who has undergone LTx and assure that the appropriate indicated childhood vaccines were received and if not, develop a plan for catch up vaccination. Many children have not received the expected immunizations based on their age at the time of LTx due to illness and other factors.[2] For many years, the recommendation was that LTx recipients should only receive nonlive virus vaccines as there was a concern for the risk of infection with live and attenuated vaccines (ie, oral polio; measles, mumps, and rubella [MMR], and Varicella [VZV]) in the face of chronic immunosuppression. Although this remains a common recommendation, there is evidence for safety of MMR and VZV vaccines in children who have undergone LTx and some centers will recommend these vaccines in select patients. Recommendations for specific vaccines follow.

Diphtheria, Pertussis, and Tetanus and Inactivated Poliovirus Vaccines

Due to the risk of polio from the oral vaccine, only inactivated poliovirus vaccine (IPV) is recommended for children who have undergone LTx. Data from several studies suggest that diphtheria, pertussis, and tetanus (DPT) and IPV vaccination rates are low in children who have undergone LTx (44%).[2] Importantly, the response rates as determined by IgG antibodies are greater than 85% in those who have been vaccinated. Thus, the focus for DPT and polio virus vaccination should be assuring primary or catch up vaccination. No further testing is indicated for individuals who have received these vaccines.

Hepatitis B Virus

Vaccination against the hepatitis B virus (HBV) is recommended for all children. In children who have undergone LTx, subsequent infection with HBV is felt to have a risk of significant morbidity and mortality. Children who have not received the HBV vaccine should be vaccinated. In children who have been vaccinated against HBV prior to LTx, up to 35% will not have protective levels of anti-HBs (heptatitis B) antibody (>10 IU/ml). Thus, children should have their anti-HBs AB status determined and those who have low titers should receive 2 doses of HBV vaccine.

Hepatitis A Virus

Vaccination against the hepatitis A virus (HAV) is also recommended for all children. Infection with HAV can lead to serious complications in LTx recipients. Since many children receive their orthotopic liver transplant prior to 1 year of age, they will not have received the HAV vaccine. Those who receive the vaccine after LTx may have a low response rate (25% to 40%).[2] Regardless, HAV vaccination should be administered if indicated as it is safe. There are no guidelines for checking anti-HAV AB titers after vaccination. Given the potential low response to the vaccine, you should assume that immunity may not be adequate in the face of an HAV exposure, and appropriate immunoprophylaxis should be administered if immunity cannot be assured by testing for anti-HAV IgG.

Varicella

The VZV infection can lead to significant complications in immunocompromised individuals. In children vaccinated prior to LTx, response rates range from 25% to 80% with waning immunity. In addition, given the large percentage of children transplanted before 1 year of age, up to 30% to 40% will not have received the VZV.[2] Vaccination with live, attenuated virus vaccines like varicella after liver transplantation is controversial. Limited studies have demonstrated good seroconversion rates of 75% to 90% with more frequent transient rashes. Primary care providers should check with the transplant center for their specific recommendations. Given the availability of immunoprophylaxis with Varicella-Zoster immune globulin (when available) and acyclovir, some centers recommend against VZV vaccination following LTx.

Measles, Mumps, and Rubella

Similar to VZV, many children do not receive the MMR vaccination prior to LTx.[2] In those who do, protective immunity seems to be good. There have been limited studies of the safety and efficacy of MMR in children after liver transplantation. These studies suggest that, in children on lower doses of immunosuppression, the MMR vaccination can lead to protective immunity.[3] As with VZV, primary care providers should check with the transplant center for its specific recommendations.

Pneumococcus

Invasive *Pneumococcal* disease is up to 6 times more frequent in pediatric solid organ transplant recipients. The *Pneumococcal* vaccine has been studied in pediatric LTx recipients and found to be safe and immunogenic, although with somewhat lower titers compared to controls. Given the higher risk of infection, children who have undergone LTx and have not received the *Pneumococcal* vaccination should be vaccinated.

Other Vaccines

The hemophilus influenzae B vaccine has been studied in renal transplant recipients and was found safe and effective, but has not been studied in LTx. Similarly, the meningococcal and human papilloma virus (HPV) vaccines have not been studied in LTx recipients. HPV infection is more common in immunocompromised individuals. Given the general safety of these vaccines, they should be considered for children and adolescents on a similar schedule to normal children. Some pediatric LTx recipients will have undergone a splenectomy. This is more common in multivisceral transplant recipients. In this case, these children should be assessed for immune response to pneumococcus and meningococcus.

Influenza

All children who have received a liver transplant should receive an annual injectable influenza vaccination as long as they do not have a contraindication (ie, egg allergy). At present live, attenuated influenza vaccination is not recommended. Immunocompromised patients are at increased risk for complications with influenza infections. The response rates to an inactive influenza vaccination have been shown to be equivalent to the general population.

Ongoing Health Maintenance Issues

There are several issues that should be part of ongoing assessment that can improve the long-term outcome following LTx.

Screen for Adherence

Rates of nonadherence to medications or clinic visits in pediatric LTx recipients is high and has been reported to range from 10% to 70%. Risk factors for nonadherence in pediatric and adolescent liver transplant patients are psychological distress, the functional status of their families, and the impact of immunosuppressive side effects on their physical appearance. No single approach has been shown to be effective, but questioning about adherence should be part of routine health maintenance visits.[4]

Screen for Hypertension

Hypertension is a common complication following LTx. The majority of patients experience hypertension in the first 1 to 2 years following liver transplantation, likely related to calcineurin inhibitor therapy and steroid use. While hypertension resolves in many of these patients as medications are reduced over time, approximately 13% of long-term surviving patients currently require antihypertensive therapy.

Post LTx, 25% to 50% of patients have a blood pressure in the >95th percentile for 1 to 5 years of age. Hypertension is primarily related to calcineurin inhibitor therapy. Assessment of renal function is indicated when hypertension is discovered with a serum creatinine and urinalysis. Treatment should be individualized but focuses on reduction of calcineurin inhibitor doses when feasible and calcium channel blockers and angiotensin converting enzyme inhibitors.

Screen for Renal Disease

Similar to hypertension and likely related, renal disease is a common complication following LTx. Anywhere from 10% to 25% of children who have undergone LTx will have significant renal dysfunction defined as a glomerular filtration rate (GFR) of less than 90 mL/min/1.73 M2 body surface area. In the primary care setting, urinalysis and serum creatinine are reasonable screening tests, but these tests underestimate renal dysfunction and many transplant centers perform measured GFR testing.

Be Alert for Potential Food Allergies

Food allergies are emerging with more frequency and are very common in children who have undergone LTx occurring in up to 40% to 50% of young recipients with severe allergies with anaphylaxis common. Screening questions for food allergies should be part of routine health maintenance and if suspicious of food allergy, refer to an allergist for evaluation and management.

Screen for Hyperlipidemia

Hyperlipidemia is common following LTx. At 10 years post LTx, 26% of pediatric recipients have hypertriglyceridemia and 20% hypercholesterolemia. Diabetes (generally type 2) is found in up to 10% of children 10 years post LTx. However, obesity is less frequent in this population, even among those on long-term steroids.[5]

Screen for School Performance and Learning Issues

School performance issues are common in children who have undergone LTx. Approximately 25% are reported to have learning issues[5] and may benefit from early interventions.

Counsel for Skin Cancer Risk

In long-term survivors following LTx, nonmelanoma skin cancer and post-transplant lymphoproliferative disease (PTLD) are the most common cancers with an incidence of 1% to 4%. PTLD is more common in childhood while skin cancer seems to begin to occur in adulthood. PTLD management is an important part of the transplant center monitoring but skin cancer risk reduction should begin in the pediatric age group. Consistent use of sunscreen is recommended for LTx recipients. Warts are the most common skin disorder in children who have undergone liver transplantation.

References

1. Kamath BM, Olthoff KM. Liver transplantation in children: update 2010. *Pediatr Clin North Am*. 2010;57:401-414.
2. Diana A, Posfay-Barbe KM, Belli DC, Siegrist CA. Vaccine-induced immunity in children after orthotopic liver transplantation: a 12-yr review of the Swiss national reference center. *Pediatr Transplant*. 2007;11:31-37.
3. Khan S, Erlichman J, Rand EB. Live virus immunization after orthotopic liver transplantation. *Pediatr Transplant*. 2006;10:78-82.
4. Kaufman M, Shemesh E, Benton T. The adolescent transplant recipient. *Pediatr Clin North Am*. 2010;57:575-592.
5. Ng VL, Alonso EM, Bucuvalas JC, et al. Health status of children alive 10 years after pediatric liver transplantation performed in the US and Canada: report of the studies of pediatric liver transplantation experience. *J Pediatr*. 2011;160:820-826.

SECTION VI

DISORDERS OF
THE PANCREAS

CONGENITAL SCREENING FOR CYSTIC FIBROSIS IS NOW THE ROUTINE IN MANY STATES. ARE THERE STILL CLINICAL SCENARIOS THAT CAN BE SEEN IN PRACTICE THAT WARRANT SUSPICION FOR CYSTIC FIBROSIS?

Tanja Gonska, MD

Newborn screening (NBS) for cystic fibrosis (CF) is based on the detection of increased levels of immune reactive trypsinogen (IRT), which is a marker of pancreatic inflammation. Each country or province has established its own screening algorithm and determines its own IRT cutoff either as absolute level or as a pre-set percentile at which point a second tier test is added to increase the specificity of the screen. Commonly, a second IRT measure or molecular analysis for the most common *cystic fibrosis transmembrane regulator (CFTR)* mutations is used as the second test. Once a newborn is screened positive, he or she will be referred to a CF center for confirmatory sweat testing, as the sweat test is still the diagnostic gold standard.[1]

The threshold for these laboratory tests is chosen to make NBS for CF highly sensitive (>95%). In return, most established NBS programs will identify a large number of heterozygote carriers as false positive screened infants. Thus, one may claim that it is highly likely that all infants with CF are identified on NBS. However, little data exist about the absolute numbers of screened newborns who have false negative NBS and who later in life are identified as having CF. While NBS started 20 to 30 years ago in some countries and a few states within the United States, it was not until recently that CF centers started to capture the numbers of false positive and false negative NBS infants. Early reports suggest that the number of false negative-screened CF patients may reach up to 8% of all identified CF patients; however, in many countries or states, screening programs have not started until recently. Thus, many children who are born before NBS will still need to be diagnosed conventionally.

So yes, you still have to be aware of CF to maintain the ability to recognize CF symptoms and to diagnose CF. Any child presenting with the following clinical scenarios should alert you to think of CF in your differential diagnosis:

- Recurrent or chronic sinopulmonary symptoms
- Nasal polyposis
- Failure to thrive due to maldigestion
- Acute recurrent or chronic pancreatitis
- Meconium ileus or distal intestinal obstruction syndrome
- Rectal prolapse
- Salt loss syndrome
- Chronic metabolic alkalosis
- Hypoalbuminemia in infancy
- Acrodermatitis enteropathica
- Prolonged neonatal jaundice
- Chronic liver disease or acute liver failure in infancy

In these cases, a sweat test with determination of the sweat chloride concentration is the recommended first line test.[1] You may add molecular analysis if the sweat test is positive or if your clinical suspicion for CF is high. It is important to remember that molecular testing has its own diagnostic pitfalls due to the existence of >1800 *CFTR* mutations and the fact that only a subset of these are known to be CF-disease causing. On the other hand, in rare cases and with certain *CFTR* mutations, sweat chloride concentrations can be false negative.

Besides the CF infant missed with NBS, you have to be aware of a new group of patients presenting for CF diagnosis who will increasingly need our attention and who will replace the classic CF infant in the near future. Over the last decade, more and more adolescents and adults have been diagnosed with CF. These patients present differently than the classic CF infant and commonly exhibit symptoms in CF-affected organs without demonstrating the full clinical picture of CF disease. Three major forms of clinical presentation have been linked to a CF diagnosis at this later age of presentation.

You may encounter older children or adolescents who present with chronic sinopulmonary disease without any other signs of systemic disease. These patients may present with recurrent nasal polyposis, chronic or recurrent bronchitis, recurrent pneumonia, and/or haemoptysis. Chest images frequently find bronchiectasis or other structural abnormalities in consequence to the chronic lung disease. Early establishment of a diagnosis and therapy is essential to prevent further progression of lung disease.[2]

Other patients may present with acute recurrent or chronic pancreatitis at an older age. These patients are pancreatic sufficient and present with or without a lung phenotype. While longitudinal data about the risk of developing lung disease in these patients are missing, a CF diagnosis should be established early to allow regular monitoring and therapeutic intervention.[3,4]

The last, large group consists of men who present to urology or fertility clinics with infertility and for whom further evaluation detects obstructive azoospermia due to congenital absence of vas deferens (CBAVD). CBAVD is present in almost all CF patients. Interestingly, about 90% of men with CBAVD carry at least one *CFTR* mutation and about 50% carry 2 *CFTR* mutations; not all of these men will meet criteria for establishing a CF diagnosis. These patients are generally lung healthy at the time of assessment and little is known about their long-term risk of developing lung disease. Thus, similar to the scenarios above, establishing a CF diagnosis and regular follow-up provides the opportunity for early intervention.[4,5]

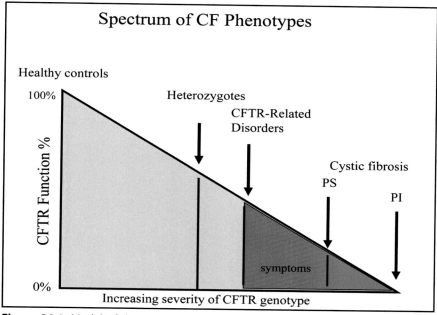

Figure 24-1. Model of the view on CF as a spectrum of disease with asymptomatic healthy controls and heterozygotes on one side of the spectrum, pancreatic sufficient (CFPS) and insufficient (CFPI) CF patients on the other side; patients with a CFTR-related disorder range in between. Patients with a CFTR-related disorder are patients presenting with chronic sinopulmonary symptoms, acute recurrent or chronic pancreatitis, as well as obstructive azoospermia.

For some of these patients, a CF diagnosis will be established following careful diagnostic evaluation.[1] Some of the patients presenting with the disease in one CF-affected organ may actually exhibit some degree of *CFTR* dysfunction but do not strictly fit the diagnostic criteria for CF. These patients are newly categorized as having a *CFTR*-related disorder (Figure 24-1).

Molecular analysis may show 0, 1, or 2 *CFTR* mutations. However, in contrast to CF, one or both mutations are not proven CF-causing mutations. Functional rather than genetic testing is helpful to establish or rule out a diagnosis for CF or a *CFTR*-related disorder with the sweat test serving as the recommended first line test. While a CF diagnosis is established following a sweat chloride concentration ≥60 mmol/L, a *CFTR*-related disorder is based on borderline sweat test results with sweat chloride concentrations ranging between 40 to 59 mmol/L. Additional adjunctive tests, such as nasal potential difference measurements performed in specialized CF diagnostic centers, may be required to help distinguish between CF and a *CFTR*-related disorder.

Both patients, those with CF and those with a *CFTR*-related disorder, should undergo complete clinical work-up to assess the degree of various organ involvement, particular with focus on the pulmonary and gastrointestinal tract. Furthermore, since patients with a *CFTR*-related disorder may suffer from lung disease that is equally severe compared to those with a confirmed CF diagnosis, management and therapy should follow the current recommendations for the treatment of CF disease in specialized CF centers.[2]

References

1. Farrell PM, Rosenstein BJ, White TB, et al. Cystic Fibrosis Foundation. Guidelines for diagnosis of cystic fibrosis in newborns through older adults: Cystic Fibrosis Foundation consensus report. *J Pediatr.* 2008;153(2):S4-S14.
2. Gonska T, Choi P, Stephenson A, et al. Role of cystic fibrosis transmembrane conductance regulator (CFTR) in patients with chronic sinopulmonary disease. *Chest.* Epub ahead of print.
3. Bishop MD, Freedman SD, Zielenski J, et al. The cystic fibrosis transmembrane conductance regulator gene and ion channel function in patients with idiopahic pancreatitis. *Hum Genet.* 2005;118(3-4):372-381.
4. Ooi CY, Dorfman R, Cipolli M, et al. Type of CFTR mutation determines risk of pancreatitis in patients with cystic fibrosis. *Gastroenterology.* 2011;140(1):153-161.
5. Wilschanski M, Dupuis A, Ellis L, et al. Mutations in the cystic fibrosis transmembrane regulator gene and in vivo transepithelial potentials. *Am J Respir Crit Care Med.* 2006;174(7):787-794.

25

WHAT CAUSES RECURRENT PANCREATITIS IN CHILDREN?

Narayanan Venkatasubramani, MBBS, MD and
Steven L. Werlin, MD

A 7-year-old boy is brought to your office with abdominal pain and vomiting. You suspect pancreatitis based on abdominal examination, and laboratory results confirm pancreatitis as demonstrated by elevated amylase and lipase. Further history reveals that the patient had 2 similar episodes of pancreatitis 1 year ago with spontaneous resolution. The parents ask you the following questions:

- What causes repeated episodes of pancreatitis?

- What investigations should be done to identify the cause of recurrent pancreatitis?

- What is the follow-up care for a patient with recurrent pancreatitis?

This chapter will discuss the etiology and a simplified diagnostic approach to the child with acute recurrent pancreatitis (ARP) or chronic pancreatitis (CP) as there are no published guidelines for the management of ARP and CP in children. In adults, ARP is defined as 2 or more separate documented episodes of acute pancreatitis presenting with abdominal pain and at least 3-fold increased serum amylase or lipase and/or imaging changes suggestive of acute pancreatitis. CP is defined as recurrent episodes of pancreatitis associated with pancreatic duct abnormalities such as dilatation, strictures, intraductal plugs containing calculi, or pancreatic insufficiency. There has been a sharp increase in diagnosis of acute pancreatitis over the last decade due to both an increase in frequency and awareness among the general pediatrician and emergency room physicians. The incidence estimate suggests that there are about 11,000 American children who present with acute pancreatitis each year with an inpatient cost alone of $200 million per year. Most children with acute pancreatitis recover uneventfully without recurrence or sequelae. However, approximately 10% to 20% of pediatric patients develop ARP or progress to CP. These patients may need multiple hospital admissions for the treatment of acute episodes and are at high risk for developing exocrine pancreatic insufficiency, diabetes mellitus, and pancreatic cancer. Hence, it is important to identify the causes of recurrent pancreatitis to prevent the progression of pancreatic duct injury and avoid further complications when possible.

The most common symptom of ARP is localized or generalized abdominal pain followed by nausea and/or vomiting. Other symptoms are jaundice, guarding, and irritability in infants and toddlers. The mean age for the onset of clinical symptoms in the initial episode of ARP is 5 years (ranging 9 months to 15 years). A gap between the onset of clinical symptoms and diagnosis of ARP may be as long as 9 years. In some patients, the delay is due to the nonspecificity of

Table 25-1
Causes and Evaluation of Acute Recurrent Pancreatitis/ Chronic Pancreatitis in Children

	Possible Diagnosis	*Investigation*
Jaundice ↑ Liver function tests	Gallstones Choledochal cyst Pancreas divisum, APBJ Trauma	Ultrasound abdomen MRCP ± secretin
Hypertension, hypothyroidism	Hypercalcemia Hypertriglyceridemia	Calcium, PTH, BUN, creatinine, TFT, TG lipoprotein profile
Medications	Valproate 6-mercaptopurine/ azathioprine Chemotherapy	Discontinuation
Family history of autoimmune disease	Autoimmune	IgG4, rheumatoid factor, anti-nuclear antibody
Family history of pancreatitis or pancreatic cancer	Hereditary pancreatitis	PRSS1 gene analysis SPINK1
Recurrent chest infection or poor growth	CF	CFTR gene analysis
All other investigations are negative	Idiopathic Sphincter of Oddi dysfunction CD IBD Organic acidemia	ERCP ± sphincterotomy and stent placement

APBJ: anomalous pancreaticobiliary junction; CF: cystic fibrosis; CD: celiac disease; IBD: inflammatory bowel disease; MRCP: magnetic resonance cholangiopancreatography; PTH: parathormone; BUN: blood urea nitrogen; TFT: thyroid function test; TG: triglycerides; PRSS1: cationic trypsinogen; SPINK1: trypsin inhibitor; CFTR: cystic fibrosis transmembrane regulator; ERCP: endoscopic retrograde cholangiopancreatography.

symptoms. ARP should be considered in the diagnostic process of pediatric patients with a history of recurrent vomiting, nausea, abdominal pain, or diarrhea as many of these patients are mistakenly diagnosed with viral gastroenteritis and further evaluation is not performed.

What Are the Causes of Acute Recurrent and Chronic Pancreatitis in Children?

The etiologies of ARP and CP in children are summarized in Table 25-1. The most common causes of ARP and CP in children have been thought to be gallstones, structural abnormalities, trauma, metabolic, and drug toxicity.[1] However, in a large study of patients with ARP/CP of all ages, etiology could not be found in 51% of patients. Improved imaging techniques and genetic testing have improved the ability to diagnose the etiology in children previously thought to have idiopathic disease.

How Do You Evaluate a Child With Acute Recurrent Pancreatitis and Chronic Pancreatitis?

Initial evaluation may be done by a pediatrician in the hospital setting and referral made to a pediatric gastroenterologist, pediatric surgeon, or other subspecialist based on the etiology of ARP and CP. As with most conditions, a detailed history is important to identify the underlying etiology. Some of the key points in the history include a medication review, a family history of pancreatitis, cystic fibrosis (CF), autoimmune disease, pancreatic cancer, recent or remote trauma (eg, falling on a bicycle handle bar), or infection. You should obtain a complete blood cell count, liver function tests, gamma-glutamyl transferase (GGT), creatinine, blood urea nitrogen (BUN), calcium, and fasting triglycerides. We recommend obtaining an abdominal ultrasound as the initial imaging modality to identify choledochal cysts, gallstones, and cholecystitis without radiation. Computed tomography is not needed to evaluate pancreatitis on initial presentation unless the diagnosis is unclear or the clinical condition deteriorates with a suspicion of pancreatic necrosis. Initial management is based on the identification of a particular etiology. We outline a management approach practiced by the pediatric gastroenterologists at our institution in Figure 25-1.

MEDICATION

First and foremost, it is important to review the full medication history as many medications can cause pancreatitis; the most common are valproic acid, 6-mercaptopurine/azathioprine, diuretics, and chemotherapeutic agents, especially L-asparaginase. These medications should be discontinued as severe morbidity and mortality can occur if continued after an episode of pancreatitis.

GENETIC CAUSES

If there is a family history of pancreatitis or CF, a genetic etiology of ARP and CP should be considered. This entails further evaluation that will be discussed later in the chapter.

METABOLIC CAUSES

Patients with hypercalcemia should be evaluated for hyperparathyroidism and renal failure. Hypertriglyceridemia can cause pancreatitis if the fasting triglycerides levels are more than 1000 and unlikely if the levels are below 500. If the patient has hypertriglyceridemia, it is important to measure thyroid function and obtain a lipoprotein profile analysis. If there is hypercalcemia or fasting hypertriglyceridemia, the patient should be referred to an endocrinologist for further evaluation.

ANATOMIC ABNORMALITIES

If the initial ultrasound shows gallstones, surgery consultation should be obtained and laproscopic cholecystectomy should be performed before discharge to prevent recurrence of pancreatitis. Endoscopic retrograde cholangiopancreatography (ERCP) is recommended before cholecystectomy if the patient has cholangitis or severe gallstone pancreatitis. If the ultrasound is normal, then the patient should be referred to a pediatric gastroenterologist for further evaluation. Typically, a

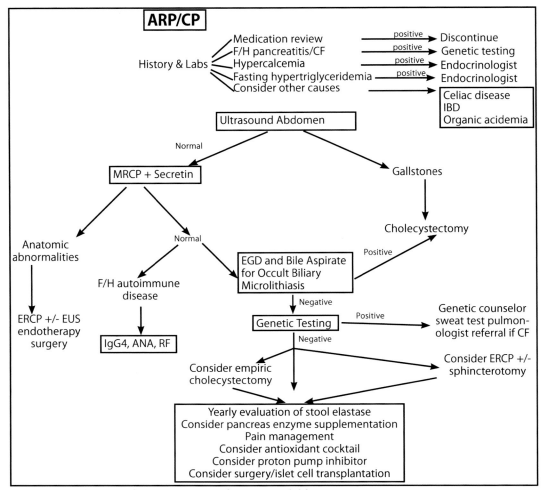

Figure 25-1. Algorithm for management of ARP/CP in children.

pediatric gastroenterologist will order magnetic resonance imaging of the pancreas (to evaluate the parenchymal architecture) and MRCP with IV secretin stimulation. Secretin distends the pancreatic ducts and allows better visualization of the ductal abnormalities such as pancreas divisum and anomalous pancreatico-biliary junction (APBJ).

If the MRCP demonstrates an anatomical abnormality or if there is evidence of CP, such as pancreatic duct dilatation, calcification, or atrophy, then an ERCP and/or endoscopic ultrasound (EUS) should be obtained and endotherapy considered. Pancreas divisum is a congenital defect wherein the majority of pancreatic tissue drains through the small dorsal pancreatic duct of Santorini. While this is seen in approximately 10% of the normal population, many patients with ARP improve symptomatically after endoscopic dorsal duct sphincterotomy and stent placement. APBJ results from malunion of the main pancreatic and common bile ducts allowing reflux of pancreatic secretions into the biliary tract that may result in gallstones, choledochal cyst, and recurrent attacks of pancreatitis. These patients need surgery and careful surveillance for cholangiocarcinoma.

If the MRCP and the metabolic laboratory results are normal, then we perform an upper gastrointestinal endoscopy with duodenal aspirate for occult biliary microlithiasis. When microlithiasis is found, the patient is referred for cholecystectomy. If there is no microlithiasis, then the patient is labeled as "idiopathic" recurrent pancreatitis. Some centers perform empiric cholecystectomy in these patients. Alternatively, an ERCP with or without EUS and possible sphincterotomy and stent placement for possible sphincter of Oddi dysfunction can be considered.[2]

AUTOIMMUNE CAUSES

If there is a strong family history of autoimmune disease or imaging studies show an enlarged pancreas with diffuse or segmental irregularity and narrowing of the pancreatic duct, a diagnosis of autoimmune pancreatitis should be considered. Autoimmune pancreatitis is very rare in children. Serum IgG4 (Immunoglobulin G4), antinuclear antibody, and rheumatoid factor should be measured. Treatment is with steroids. A pancreatic biopsy may be helpful in cases of diagnostic uncertainty.

IDIOPATHIC

Approximately 50% of pediatric patients do not have an identified etiology in spite of the above investigations. A genetic etiology should be considered if there is a family history of pancreatitis, CF, and/or other etiologies of ARP are negative. After a detailed discussion with the parents, gene mutations in the *cystic fibrosis transmembrane regulator (CFTR)*, PRSS1, and SPINK1 genes should be sought.[3] If a mutation is found, these patients should be referred to a genetic counselor. Identifying a genetic mutation in these patients can have other important clinical implications since some mutations are associated with an increased risk of pancreatic insufficiency and pancreatic cancer. These patients are more likely to advance to CP and may not benefit from empiric cholecystectomy or sphincterotomy.[3] Patients with mutations in the *CFTR* gene should be evaluated for CF. Sweat tests may be normal in atypical *CFTR*-related pancreatitis. Other rare causes of ARP include celiac disease, inflammatory bowel disease, organic acidemia, and other metabolic disorders.

What Is the Follow-Up for Patients With Acute Recurrent Pancreatitis and Chronic Pancreatitis?

Patients with ARP and CP need to have yearly evaluations of pancreatic function either by stool elastase or 72-hour stool fat collection. These patients need to be supplemented with pancreatic enzymes when maldigestion is present (see Question 27). The majority of patients with CP will need referral to a pain clinic for treatment of debilitating pain. Some patients may get relief from pain with a trial of pancreas enzyme supplements and/or antioxidants (ie, selenium, beta-carotene, vitamin C, vitamin E, and methionine). Tricyclic antidepressants are useful both by altering central-pain perception and by treating concomitant depression. If conservative treatment fails, the patient may require endotherapy in the form of sphincterotomy and stent placement. Partial pancreatic resection or pancreatectomy with islet cell transplantation is indicated when all of the above therapies are unsuccessful. Patients need to be educated about the avoidance of alcohol and smoking as it increases the risk of pancreatitis and later pancreatic cancer.

References

1. Werlin SL, Kugathasan S, Frautschy BC. Pancreatitis in children. *J Pediatr Gastroenterol Nutr*. 2003;37(5):591-595.
2. Papachristou G, Topazian M. Idiopathic recurrent pancreatitis: an EUS-based management approach. *Gastrointest Endosc*. 2011;73(6):1155-1157.

3. Sultan M, Werlin S, Venkatasubramani N. Genetic prevalence and characteristics in children with recurrent pancreatitis. *J Pediatr Gastroenterol Nutr*. 2012;54(5):645-650.

Review Articles

Gelrud A, Sheth S, Banerjee S, et al. Analysis of cystic fibrosis gene production (CFTR) function in patients with pancreas divisum and recurrent acute pancreatitis. *Am J Gastroenterol*. 2004;99(8):1557-1562.

QUESTION 26

EXOCRINE PANCREATIC INSUFFICIENCY IS UNUSUAL IN PEDIATRICS. ARE THERE CLINICAL CONDITIONS OTHER THAN CYSTIC FIBROSIS THAT CAN CAUSE PANCREATIC INSUFFICIENCY?

Kathy D. Chen, MD and Sohail Z. Husain, MD

Although cystic fibrosis (CF) is the leading cause of pancreatic insufficiency (PI) in children, there are several other pediatric syndromes that can cause PI (Table 26-1).

Signs and Symptoms of Pancreatic Insufficiency

Pancreatic insufficiency (PI) is defined as the inability to properly digest food due to a lack of digestive enzymes made by the pancreas. The primary symptom of PI is steatorrhea, or the presence of excess fat in the stool resulting from the malabsorption of dietary fat. Patients or their families will often describe seeing greasy stools with orange droplets. The stools are found to float in toilet water, and they may have a film of oil surrounding them. They may be bulky and loose, which can cause patients to come in with complaints of diarrhea. Patients with PI often come in for an evaluation of failure to thrive. It is important to recognize that steatorrhea does not equate to PI. Several other conditions are accompanied by steatorrhea, including enteritis (such as from celiac disease) and cholestasis.

WHY DOES PANCREATIC INSUFFICIENCY CAUSE STEATORRHEA?

Over 85% of the pancreas is made up of exocrine components: acinar cells and duct cells. Together, the 2 cell types coordinate the regulated release and flow of pancreatic juice into the intestinal lumen. Acinar cells primarily synthesize, store, and secrete pancreatic enzymes, whereas duct cells secrete fluid and bicarbonate. Among the different enzymes in pancreatic juice, pancreatic lipase is necessary for the lipolysis of triglycerides in dietary fat into their nonesterified form as free fatty acids. Although lipases make up only about 2% of the pancreatic enzymes

Table 26-1

Causes of Pancreatic Insufficiency in Children

Disease	OMIM	Gene/Locus	Comments
CF	219700	CFTR	Most common
SDS	260400	SBDS	Hematologic abnormalities and malignancies
Johanson-Blizzard syndrome (JBS)	243800	UBR1	Nasal alar hypoplasia, congenital deafness
Pearson marrow-pancreas syndrome (PMPS)	557000	mtDNA	Refractory anemia in infancy
Pancreatic agenesis	260370	IPF1	Both endocrine and exocrine PI
Congenital lipase deficiency	614338	PNLIP	Steatorrhea, but usually without FTT
Congenital enterokinase deficiency	226200	PRSS7	Protein malabsorption; no steatorrhea
Syndrome of PI, dyserythropoietic anemia, calvarial hyperostosis	612714	COX4I2	Steatorrhea, FTT, anemia
Pancreatic and cerbellar agenesis	609069	PTF1A	Diabetes mellitus, cerebellar agenesis
Chronic pancreatitis (CP)			PI seen mainly in adults
After extensive pancreatectomy, or rarely, pancreatic obliteration after a severe, necrotic bout of acute pancreatitis			

OMIM: Online Mendelian Inheritance in Man. CF: cystic fibrosis; SDS: Shwachman-Diamond syndrome; JBS: Johanson-Blizzard syndrome; PMPS: Pearson marrow-pancreas syndrome; PI: pancreatic insufficiency; CP: chronic pancreatitis; FTT: failure to thrive.

load, their reduction leads to the symptoms of steatorrhea during PI. The lipase output, however, needs to drop to less than 10% below normal levels in order to develop fat malabsorption. These observations not only demonstrate the large reserve capacity of lipase secretion by the pancreas, but they also suggest that nonpancreatic sources of lipase, such as gastric lipase or in breastfed infants, carboxyester lipase from breast milk can contribute to lipolysis.

Cystic Fibrosis

In children, CF is the most common cause of PI and, for this reason, always needs to be considered in the differential diagnosis of PI. The autosomal recessive defect in the *cystic fibrosis*

Table 26-2
Diagnosis of Shwachman-Diamond Syndrome

- Clinical diagnosis consists of a combination of hematological cytopenia of any given lineage (most often neutropenia) and exocrine pancreas dysfunction.
- Additional supportive evidence may come from bone abnormalities, behavioral problems, or a first-degree family member diagnosed with SDS.
- Molecular testing for bi-allelic SBDS gene mutation is recommended, along with genetic counseling.

---

transmembrane regulator (CFTR) occurs with an incidence of 1 in 2500 in White patients. Two-thirds of patients with classic CF will develop signs of PI as infants, whereas, another one-fifth of patients (totaling about 85% of all classic CF cases) will have a progressive loss of pancreatic function by 3 years of age. The prevailing notion for the development of PI in CF is that the loss of *CFTR* causes reduced ion and fluid transport into the pancreatic duct, which leads to ductal plugging and the eventual destruction, mostly in utero, of the exocrine pancreas.

Shwachman-Diamond Syndrome

Beyond CF though, there are several other causes of PI. Shwachman-Diamond syndrome (SDS) is the second most common syndrome of PI, occurring with a frequency of about one-twentieth that of CF. SDS was first described in 1964 by Drs. Shwachman, Diamond, and Bodian as a triad of PI, bone marrow dysfunction, and short stature. Unlike CF, there is no ethnic preference. In 2003, the autosomal recessive disorder was linked in about 90% of SDS patients to mutations in a single gene, dubbed the Shwachman–Bodian–Diamond syndrome (SBDS) gene. The SBDS gene encodes for a protein involved in the biogenesis and transport of the large mammalian ribosomal subunit. Owing to their function in synthesizing massive amounts of pancreatic enzymes, pancreatic acinar cells are relatively more vulnerable to translational impairment caused by the loss of function mutations in SBDS. This may explain why almost all SDS patients have PI. Histologically, there is replacement of acinar cells by fatty infiltration, whereas the islets and ducts are largely intact. The lipomatosis and atrophy of pancreatic parenchyma can be appreciated by computed tomography scan or magnetic resonance imaging.

In contrast to CF cases, patients with SDS have low-serum pancreatic enzymes at birth, including serum trypsinogen. Other clinical findings associated with SDS include hematological dysfunction with neutropenia as the most common sign, followed by thrombocytopenia. Patients can have skeletal abnormalities, usually presenting with metaphyseal dysplasia in the long bones and costochondral junctions. Patients can also have neurodevelopmental defects and abnormalities involving the liver, kidneys, teeth, or brain.

Based on a 2011 draft consensus statement, the diagnosis of SDS requires the combined presence of PI and a hematological cytopenia of any given lineage (Table 26-2). PI can be diagnosed by demonstrating reduced levels of pancreatic enzymes in serum or stool (eg, a low fecal elastase-1). Tests that would support the diagnosis of SDS but require corroboration include an abnormal 72-hour fecal fat analysis, reduced levels of at least 2 fat-soluble vitamins, or evidence of pancreatic lipomatosis. Additional supportive evidence of SDS includes identification of bony abnormalities,

Figure 26-1. Infant with JBS, who had PI, severe developmental delay, and characteristic hypoplasia or aplasia of the nasal wings.

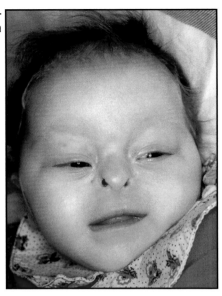

behavioral disturbances, or a family history of SDS. Genetic testing for SDS is clinically available and can be used to make a molecular diagnosis of the disease. In fact, the 2011 consensus group advised testing most or all suspected cases for mutations in the SBDS gene. There are, however, several caveats in the interpretation of the genetic results, including a 10% false-negative rate. In such cases, a strong clinical suspicion is necessary to guide the diagnosis and other causes of PI need to be carefully examined. Genetic counseling is recommended alongside genetic testing for SDS.

The management of PI in patients with SDS is similar to that of CF, which primarily utilizes pancreatic enzyme replacement therapy (PERT) and fat-soluble vitamin supplementation. Notably, half of SDS patients outgrow the need for PERT by 4 years of age, although some level of PI remains. Readers are referred to the consensus statement for details of additional testing at diagnosis and at follow-up for the nonpancreatic features of SDS, such as hematological malignancy surveillance and skeletal interventions. Although prospective data are lacking, patients with SDS probably have normal life expectancy.

Johanson-Blizzard Syndrome

Johanson-Blizzard syndrom (JBS), first described in 1967, consists of PI, severe developmental delay, and characteristic hypoplasia or aplasia of the nasal wings (Figure 26-1). There are less than a few hundred reported cases, making it rare. In 2005, the disease was linked to a loss of function mutation in the UBR1 gene that encodes an E3 ubiquitin ligase, a factor that is necessary for recognizing certain proteins destined to a cellular degradation or proteosomal pathway. UBR1 is highly expressed in pancreatic acinar cells and is, therefore, thought to be important in maintaining quality control of protein in the acinar cell. This might explain why patients with JBS are observed to have a destructive pancreatitis of intrauterine onset. In fact, PI is the most consistent clinical feature of the syndrome. The pancreas becomes replaced by fat and connective tissue. In adulthood, endocrine insufficiency may also develop. Additional clinical features include a small, beak-like nose due to aplasia or hypoplasia of the nasal alae, severe developmental delay, oligodontia, sensori-neural hearing loss, hypothyroidism, scalp defects, urogenital malformations, and congenital heart defects. Molecular testing is usually not indicated, but may be helpful in some cases.

In contrast to SDS and other syndromes associated with PI, patients with JBS do not have hematological abnormalities. Management guidelines parallel that of CF management with the use of PERT and fat-soluble vitamins.

Pearson Marrow-Pancreas Syndrome

Another rare syndrome is the Pearson marrow-pancreas syndrome (PMPS). Usually diagnosed in infancy, the syndrome is associated with PI, severe hypoplastic, macrocytic anemia, and varying degrees of other multiorgan involvement such as hepatic, renal, and neuromuscular. The hematologic defects dominate. Patients present at birth with severe, transfusion-dependent sideroblastic anemia and may also have neutropenia and thrombocytopenia. The pancreas is found to be fibrotic.

PMPS is due to deletions in mitochondrial deoxyribonucleic acid (mtDNA), which is a small chromosomal sequence, housed within mitochondria, that encodes several of the proteins and ribonucleic acid necessary for mitochondrial function. Affected individuals can be diagnosed by the above clinical picture, high serum lactate or pyruvate, and by a southern blot demonstrating mtDNA rearrangements. Treatment is supportive. Patients usually succumb to death in infancy or toddlerhood, mainly due to metabolic disorders or infections. Those who survive can manifest a phenotypic shift from a predominantly hematopoietic to a neuromuscular disorder resembling the features of another mitochondrial disease, Kearns-Sayre syndrome. The maternal inheritance pattern or phenotypic severity for disorders of mtDNA, such as PMPS, is complex. Part of the reason is that each cell in the body has several hundred mitochondria, each with its own mtDNA. Furthermore, mtDNA deletions usually occur *de novo* in the proband. Taken together, the risk of siblings of a proband being affected is very low, and even affected women have a small chance (approximately 1 in 24 births) of having an affected child. Offspring of affected men are not at risk.

Other Rare Causes of Pancreatic Insufficiency

Other rare cases of PI are caused by deficiencies in specific pancreatic enzymes or their cofactors, or global defects in pancreatic development, including congenital pancreatic lipase or colipase deficiency. Patients with the former were reported to have steatorrhea in infancy, and in one case, developed it after switching from breastfeeding to whole milk. Growth failure was not observed and the steatorrhea was effectively treated with PERT and a low-fat diet. Patients with colipase deficiency presented with steatorrhea during early childhood. Congenital enterokinase deficiency is a rare cause of PI that does not lead to steatorrhea. Patients presented with diarrhea, failure to thrive, and hypoproteinemic edema as infants. They had protein malabsorption, which is consistent with the crucial function of enterokinase (also known as enteropeptidase) along the intestinal brush border as an activator of the pancreatic protease cascade, starting with the cleavage of trypsinogen to its active form trypsin. There may be some independent activation of trypsin during adulthood that might explain why several adult patients were able to successfully wean off PERT.

Loss of function mutations in the genes encoding transcription factors that are critical for development of the pancreas, but that do not preclude fetal death, can lead to PI as well as endocrine failure. Loss of function mutations in the insulin promoter factor-1 gene are associated with the syndrome of congenital pancreatic agenesis, which results in PI, neonatal diabetes, and intrauterine growth retardation. Mutations in pancreas transcription factor 1-alpha are associated with pancreatic and cerebellar agenesis.

Finally, it is notable that CP that leads to the destruction of the pancreatic parenchyma is the most common cause of PI in the general population. However, PI in this situation takes decades to develop and is, therefore, primarily of adult onset.

Conclusion

Steatorrhea is the primary symptom of PI. But it is important to keep in mind that several other conditions, such as enteritis or cholestasis, can cause steatorrhea. Though classic CF is the most common cause of PI in children, there are several other inherited causes. SDS is the second most frequent, followed by JBS. Each of these syndromes has characteristic organ system involvement, and most have specific gene defects. A broad differential should, therefore, be considered when evaluating a child who presents with PI.

Bibliography

DiMagno E, Go VL, Summerskill WH. Relations between pancreatic enzyme outputs and malabsorption in severe pancreatic insufficiency. *N Engl J Med.* 1973;288(5):813-815.

Dror Y, Donadieu J, Koglmeier J, et al. Draft consensus guidelines for diagnosis and treatment of Shwachman-Diamond syndrome. *Ann N Y Acad Sci.* 2011;1242:40-55.

Zenker M, Mayerle J, Reis A, Lerch MM. Genetic basis and pancreatic biology of Johanson-Blizzard syndrome. *Endocrinol Metab Clin of North Am.* 2006;35(2):243-253, vii-viii.

HOW SHOULD I USE PANCREATIC ENZYMES IN CHILDREN WITH CYSTIC FIBROSIS AND OTHER CAUSES OF PANCREATIC INSUFFICIENCY?

Mark E. Lowe, MD, PhD and Douglas Lindblad, MD

Pancreatic enzyme replacement therapy (PERT) is essential for patients with pancreatic exocrine insufficiency. In children, the most common cause of pancreatic insufficiency is cystic fibrosis (CF) followed by Shwachman-Diamond syndrome (SDS) and chronic pancreatitis (CP). When caring for patients with these diagnoses, the first question we ask is whether they have pancreatic insufficiency. Of patients with CF, 10% to 15% will not have pancreatic insufficiency. Larger fractions of patients with SDS or CP will also not have pancreatic insufficiency. Although it is clear that patients with pancreatic insufficiency should be treated with PERT, there is controversy about treating patients with evidence of pancreatic disease who do not have pancreatic insufficiency even though their pancreatic function may be decreased. We generally do not prescribe PERT to patients without objective evidence of pancreatic insufficiency.

Although a history and examination can suggest pancreatic insufficiency, we do not rely on that information in making treatment decisions. Symptoms such as bulky stools or abdominal pain are not specific for pancreatic insufficiency. Poor growth is not necessarily a result of pancreatic insufficiency, although all of these symptoms should prompt you to consider pancreatic insufficiency in at-risk patient populations.

In general, we confirm the diagnosis of pancreatic insufficiency with objective testing. The most accurate method is intubation of the duodenum with timed collections. The method is rarely used since it is invasive, labor intensive, and not readily available. Some physicians collect duodenal fluid after stimulation of pancreatic secretions with secretin and cholecystokinin during upper endoscopy for determination of pancreatic enzyme levels. This method is probably helpful if normal levels are found but there are multiple reasons to find low levels apart from pancreatic insufficiency. For most patients, we prefer quantification of the coefficient of fat absorption. The 72-hour stool collection for fecal fat has lost favor in many centers because it requires careful control of dietary fat, takes 3 days, and stool collection is unpleasant for many families. In children, the adult standard of feeding meals with 100 g of fat each day is often not feasible. We have the family keep a diet history and have our dieticians calculate the dietary fat intake over the collection period. A recent study suggested that a 24-hour stool collection might be adequate but this has not been confirmed and we do not recommend its use. In some centers, 13C-mixed triglyceride

	Table 27-1
	Recommended Pancreatic Enzyme Dose in Cystic Fibrosis
Age	*Dose*
Infants	2000 to 5000 lipase units per 120 mL of formula or with each breastfeed
Four years and younger	1000 to 2500 lipase units per kg per meal
	500 lipase units per kg per snack
	Up to 10,000 lipase units per kg per day
Four years and older	500 to 2500 lipase units per kg per meal
	250 lipase units per kg per snack
	Up to 10,000 lipase units per kg per day
Adolescents and adults	Similar to above although lower doses may be adequate since fat intake per kg declines with age

breath testing is available and offers an alternative to a fecal fat collection. In recent years, we have ordered fecal elastase testing to screen patients for pancreatic insufficiency. Pancreatic elastase is stable during transit through the intestines and colon. Available tests discriminate between the human and pig enzyme allowing use even if a patient is already taking PERT. This allows you to start PERT in patients you strongly suspect have pancreatic insufficiency immediately and still perform an objective test. The diagnostic utility of fecal elastase has been validated in patients with CF and SDS. We also order fecal elastase in patients with evidence of CP although use in this patient population is less established.

In CF, there is a strong correlation between the pancreatic function (a phenotype of either pancreatic insufficiency or sufficiency) and the gene mutations (genotype) causing disease. Mutations in the *cystic fibrosis transmembrane regulator (CFTR)* gene have been classified into 2 categories: mild and severe. Patients with 2 severe mutations develop pancreatic insufficiency; for example, over 99% of those homozygous for the most common mutation, delta-F508, have pancreatic insufficiency. You should anticipate that infants and young children who carry 2 severe *CFTR* mutations will have pancreatic insufficiency. A confirmatory test, such as a pancreatic elastase measurement, can be useful and provides some additional information in this setting but is not absolutely necessary. Patients carrying one or more mild *CFTR* mutations may not have pancreatic insufficiency. In fact, many of these patients will be pancreatic sufficient and they should be tested for pancreatic insufficiency.

Once a diagnosis of pancreatic insufficiency is made, PERT should be prescribed. The goal is to normalize absorption of nutrients. Our practice is to follow the guidelines for patients with CF in prescribing PERT to all patients with pancreatic insufficiency (Table 27-1). In general, we do not prescribe doses greater than 2500 lipase units/kg unless there is evidence of fat malabsorption prior to the increase and evidence for improvement of fat absorption after increasing the dose. The timing of each dose is still not firmly established. We generally suggest taking PERT just before a meal or snack. Some physicians suggest giving part of the dose after the start of the meal and then at the end of the meal. The timing of PERT administration may need to be individualized

Table 27-2

Clinical Assessment of Nutritional Status in Patients With Pancreatic Exocrine Insufficiency

History	Weight loss or gain
	Medications
	Alcohol use in older patients
	Gastrointestinal (GI) or pancreatic surgery
	Dietary intake and restrictions
	Symptoms of nutrient intolerance (eg, diarrhea, abdominal pain, and vomiting)
	Symptoms of nutrient deficiencies (eg, hair loss, glossitis, dermatitis, and parethesias)
Anthropometry	Body weight
	Height
	Body mass index (BMI)
	Arm circumference
Biochemical tests	Plasma proteins (eg, albumin, retinal binding protein, prealbumin, and transferrin)
	Fat soluble vitamins A, D, E, and K
	Cholesterol
	Complete blood cell count (CBC) with differential
Muscle function	Strength testing

GI: gastrointestinal; BMI: body mass index; CBC: complete blood cell count.

for some patients. Older children can swallow the capsules; for younger children, PERT can be opened and the microcapsules mixed in a nonalkaline food, such as applesauce or milk. For infants, the capsules can be mixed with a small amount of expressed human milk, formula, or fruit puree and given with a spoon. Remember to educate patients to take enzymes with all fat-containing foods and drinks. If your patient is tube fed, then dosing may take trial and error. For patients on continuous feeds, lower doses may be adequate because gastric lipase may digest a larger fraction of dietary fats in this situation. Generally, PERT is provided at the start of the infusion and at the end. Some may require a dose during the infusion. If your patient is bolus fed, then give PERT at the start of the feed and remember larger doses may be required rather than needed for patients on continuous feeds.

Once you have started your patient on PERT, it is important to monitor nutritional parameters for efficacy (Table 27-2). If your patient has a poor response to therapy as manifested by persistent complaints of abdominal pain, bloating, flatus, change in stools, or by poor growth, you should consider factors that may cause these symptoms and not simply escalate the PERT dose. Your first step is to confirm that your patient takes the dose correctly and that the enzymes are stored properly (ie, avoiding exposure to cold, heat, and moisture). Next you should review the patient's diet and eating behavior. The patient may prefer higher-fat foods, have excessive juice intake, or may have a habit of grazing on food. You should then address compliance. Many factors can affect whether your patient takes his or her PERT. Toddlers can be stubborn and refuse to take the medication. Many times there are multiple caregivers in the home or the child splits time between divorced parents and doses are missed. Older children can refuse to take PERT because they are depressed, angry, or are afraid they will seem different from their peers. If your questioning has not provided a clear direction, then a trial of acid suppression is reasonable. Currently, that usually means a proton pump inhibitor, although H2-blockers can be tried. Remember that the exocrine pancreas secretes bicarbonate that is necessary for the proper dissolution of the microcapsules and release of the enzymes. Once released from the microcapsules, the enzymes, particularly pancreatic lipase, can be inactivated by an acidic environment. If the patient is already on acid suppression and still symptomatic, it is reasonable to empirically increase the PERT dose provided the current dose is below the recommended maximum. If the indicators of poor efficacy improve with changes in dosing, timing, compliance, or addition of acid suppression, then you should continue to monitor the patient.

If your patient's symptoms do not improve, you should investigate these symptoms to rule out other causes of gastrointestinal dysfunction (Table 27-3). In a patient with CF, you must remember that intestinal function is affected and that may impact on absorption of nutrients apart from digestion. Still, you need to consider other diagnoses in patients with CF and with other causes of pancreatic insufficiency. Often you will find that a thorough investigation does not provide an explanation for your patient's persistent symptoms. In that instance, you may be tempted to increase the dose of PERT. Too often that approach leads to recurrent dose escalation. Keep in mind that clinical evaluation is not specific or sensitive for efficacy of PERT. You should obtain objective evidence for steatorrhea by ordering a 72-hour fecal-fat collection or, if available to you, a 13C-mixed triglyceride breath test. If steatorrhea is present, then dose adjustment is in order.

Bibliography

Borowitz D, Durie PR, Clarke LL, et al. Gastrointestinal outcomes and confounders in cystic fibrosis. *J Pediatr Gastroenterol Nutr.* 2005;41(3):273-285.

Cystic Fibrosis Foundation; Borowitz D, Robinson KA, Rosenfeld M, et al. Cystic Fibrosis Foundation evidence-based guidelines for management of infants with cystic fibrosis. *J Pediatr.* 2009;155(suppl 6):S73-S93.

Dominguez-Munoz JE. Chronic pancreatitis and persistent steatorrhea: what is the correct dose of enzymes? *Clin Gastroenterol Hepatol.* 2011;9(7):541-546.

Wouthuyzen-Bakker M, Bodewes FA, Verkade HJ. Persistent fat malabsorption in cystic fibrosis; lessons from patients and mice. *J Cyst Fibros.* 2011;10(3):150-158.

Table 27-3

Gastrointestinal Confounders of Pancreatic Insufficiency That Will Not Respond to Increasing Pancreatic Enzyme Replacement Therapy

Diagnosis	Evaluation
Liver disease	Evidence of portal hypertension on exam, alkaline phosphatase, GGT, bilirubin panel, serum transaminases, ultrasound, and cholangiogram
Enteric infection • Parasites (Giardia in particular) • Bacteria • Pseudomembranous colitis	Stool for culture, ova and parasite and giardia antigen, *Clostridium difficile* toxin assay
Bacterial overgrowth	Breath test
Lactose intolerance	Dietary elimination trial or breath test
CD	Tissue transglutaminase-IgA, serum IgA, small bowel biopsy
Short bowel syndrome	Surgical history
Crohn's disease	CBC, erythrocyte sedimentation rate, C-reactive protein, enterography, colonoscopy with biopsy, upper endoscopy with biopsy, and capsule endoscopy
Eating disorder	History and elimination of other causes for weight loss or anorexia
Functional disorders (chronic abdominal pain, IBS)	History and directed evaluation for other causes of GI symptoms

CD: celiac disease; IBS: irritable bowel syndrome; GGT: gamma-glutamyl transferase; CBC: complete blood cell count; CRP: C-reactive protein; GI: gastrointestinal.

SECTION VII

UPPER GASTROINTESTINAL AND SMALL BOWEL TOPICS

28

CELIAC DISEASE SEEMS SO MUCH MORE COMMON. IS THIS AN EPIDEMIC?

Ivor D. Hill, MB, ChB, MD

Prior to the mid 1990s, celiac disease (CD) was regarded as being relatively rare in the United States. Since then, several studies have shown, conclusively, the condition is as common in the United States as in Europe and many other countries around the world and affects approximately 1% of the general population.[1] Today, pediatricians in general practice are diagnosing CD in ever increasing numbers. In addition, recent reports suggest the prevalence of CD in adults has increased in the past 3 decades.[2,3] Taken together, these observations might lead one to question whether there is an epidemic of CD and if so, why?

To put this into perspective, in the United States there are 2 issues that need consideration. The first is that previously CD was significantly underdiagnosed due to the lack of clinical suspicion for the condition. Health care providers are now more aware of the variable clinical manifestations of CD, and hence more likely to use serologic tests to screen for the condition. Most children with CD present with gastrointestinal (GI) manifestations, such as diarrhea, abdominal pain, or bloating and poor weight gain or weight loss, but others have constipation, nausea, and/or vomiting. These symptoms can begin at any age, may occur singly or in combination, can be continuous or intermittent, and vary in severity. CD may also present initially with non-GI features, such as isolated short stature, anemia, dental enamel defects, unexplained fatigue, or delay in onset of puberty. In addition, many children have associated conditions that put them at increased risk for CD. At risk groups include family members of a known case of CD and those with type 1 diabetes, autoimmune thyroiditis, Down syndrome, Turner syndrome, Williams syndrome, and selective IgA deficiency. Serological screening of these individuals has identified many with CD even though they are asymptomatic. Serological tests to screen for CD have also improved in the past 15 years. The identification of tissue transglutaminase (tTG) as the autoantigen in CD lead to development of tests that identify an antibody to tTG. This is highly sensitive and specific for CD and is recommended as the test of choice to identify those that require a biopsy to confirm the diagnosis.[4] In my opinion, it is this new appreciation of the varied clinical manifestations of CD, and use of tTG as a screening test, that is largely responsible for the increase in the number of patients being diagnosed with the condition in the United States.

The second issue is a probable genuine increase in the prevalence of CD. Recent studies from Finland and the United States demonstrate the prevalence of tTG-positive serology in the general population has risen significantly over the past 3 decades.[2,3] Because a positive tTG test correlates strongly with biopsy evidence for CD, this suggests the prevalence of CD is increasing. If there has been an increase in the prevalence of CD, the question is, why? The onset of CD is dependent on a genetic predisposition together with exposure to an environmental trigger, with ingestion of gluten being one essential component. Additional triggers are suspected to play a role in some cases, but these are not yet clearly identified. Changes in the genetic component of CD cannot be implicated given the relatively short time period in which this has occurred. Therefore, we must assume that any increase in the prevalence of CD is due to some change in an environmental component.

Variations in dietary practices may be one explanation. These could involve either the amount of gluten ingested or the age at which gluten is first introduced into the diet. The recent experience in Sweden where there was an "epidemic" of CD in young children from the mid 1980s to the mid 1990s supports this possibility.[5] During this time, there was a 4-fold rise in the number of young children diagnosed with CD. This coincided with a decrease in the duration of breastfeeding and an early introduction of weaning foods that were high in gluten content. Subsequent promotion of prolonged breastfeeding with a decrease in gluten content in weaning foods saw a return in the number of young children with CD to pre-epidemic levels. It remains to be seen whether prolonged breastfeeding, with introduction of smaller amounts of gluten initially, will lead to a lasting decrease in the prevalence of CD or merely delay onset of the disease until a later age.

We also know the intestinal bacterial flora plays a significant role in health and disease, and the composition of the gut microbiome has been implicated in the pathogenesis of a number of autoimmune diseases. This concept is embodied in the theory behind the "hygiene hypothesis." In simplistic terms, the postulate is that lack of early childhood exposure to infectious and parasitic agents, due in part to improvements in hygiene and liberal use of antibiotics, suppresses natural development of the immune system that increases susceptibility to autoimmune disease. The marked increase in immune-mediated disorders such as asthma, diabetes, inflammatory bowel disease, and eczema in developed nations as opposed to undeveloped countries supports this possibility. A recently published study from Finland suggests this concept plays a role in CD as well. In this study, the prevalence of CD in children living in a region of Finland was compared to that of a bordering region in Russia. There was a significantly higher rate of positive serological tests for CD in the Finish children. There were no differences between the 2 regions in regard to the frequency of the celiac-related human leukocyte antigen genotypes but there were significant differences in the socioeconomic status with those in Finland having higher levels of hygiene and lower rates of childhood infections and parasitic infestation.

Finally, any rise in the frequency of CD must not be confused with the marked increase in the number of people who claim improvements in health and well being by avoiding gluten in their diet. The gluten-free diet has, to some extent, become the new fad diet and is being followed by many celebrities and sports stars who claim beneficial effects. There is an emerging concept of an entity known as non-CD gluten sensitivity. This is used to describe individuals who have a variety of nonspecific symptoms that resolve after starting a strict gluten-free diet. These individuals often do not have positive tests for CD, or at most have only elevated antibodies to the gliadin tests that are regarded as nonspecific. Furthermore, in those who have had intestinal biopsies, there is no evidence of CD. Based on some recent reports, it seems the entity of non-CD gluten sensitivity does in fact exist, but it remains to be determined how to confirm the diagnosis and how prevalent this condition actually is. It is possible the health benefits claimed by many individuals who place themselves on a gluten-free diet are related more to the fact that they are now eating a healthy diet than to the fact they are restricting gluten.

Conclusion

The marked increase in the number of people being diagnosed with CD in the United States is predominantly due to the fact that physicians now recognize the protean manifestations of the condition and use appropriate tests to screen for it. To a lesser degree, the increase may be related to a true rise in the prevalence. The reasons for this rise in prevalence are not yet clear but presumably are related to some environmental change that precipitates disease in genetically predisposed individuals. CD should not be confused with the entity of non-CD gluten sensitivity. Distinguishing between CD, non-CD gluten sensitivity, and even wheat allergy is important as there are potentially significant prognostic and therapeutic implications.

References

1. Fasano A, Berti I, Gerarduzzi T, et al. Prevalence of celiac disease in at-risk and not at-risk groups in the United States: a large multicenter study. *Arch Int Med.* 2003;163(3):286-292.
2. Lohi S, Mustalahti K, Kaukinen K, et al. Increasing prevalence of coeliac disease over time. *Aliment Pharmacol Ther.* 2007;26(9):1217-1225.
3. Rubio-Tapia A, Kyle RA, Kaplan EL, et al. Increased prevalence and mortality in undiagnosed celiac disease. *Gastroenterology.* 2009;137(1):88-93.
4. Hill I, Dirks M, Colletti R, et al. North American Society for Pediatric Gastroenterology, Hepatology and Nutrition. Guideline for the diagnosis and treatment of celiac disease in children: recommendations of the North American Society for Pediatric Gastroenterology, Hepatology and Nutrition. *J Pediatr Gastroenterol Nutr.* 2005;40(1):1-19.
5. Ivarsson A, Persson LA, Nystrom L, et al. Epidemic of coeliac disease in Swedish children. *Acta Paediatr.* 2000;89(2):165-171.

ARE THERE GROUPS WHO ARE AT AN INCREASED RISK FOR CELIAC DISEASE THAT SHOULD BE SCREENED?

Thomas Flass, MD, MS and Edward J. Hoffenberg, MD

At present, only children with a risk factor should be screened for celiac disease (CD).

Why Not Screen All Children?

With good evidence that the incidence of CD in the United States is greater than 1 in 100, some researchers argue for uniform screening of all children. Proponents of mass screening often bring up the fact that health care providers regularly screen for far more rare diseases than CD on newborn screening. However, mainly because of uncertain natural history and absence of severe consequences of delayed diagnosis in most cases, universal screening is not cost effective or practical.[1]

The significance of seropositivity in an asymptomatic individual identified on routine screening is unclear and the benefit of early diagnosis and treatment is unproven. There are no current recommendations to do anything other than follow these patients for development of signs or symptoms of active disease. Therefore, current guidelines take the approach to not screen all children for CD and instead focus on testing those with an increased risk.

What Are the Risk Groups That Should Prompt Screening?

Traditionally, at-risk groups have been categorized as those with signs or symptoms of concern, associated conditions, or family history. Both the North American Society for Pediatric Gastroenterology, Hepatology and Nutrition (NASPGHAN)[2] and European Society for Paediatric Gastroenterology, Hepatology and Nutrition (ESPGHAN)[3] have developed

Table 29-1
Populations at Increased Genetic Risk

Risk	Prevalence (per 100 people)
Type 1 diabetes	Up to 8% to 10% with biopsy proven and 16% with positive celiac serology
Down syndrome	3.8% to 13%
Turner syndrome	4% to 8%
Williams syndrome	8% to 9%
IgA deficiency	2% to 8%
Autoimmune disease including: Thyroiditis Hepatitis	2% to 8% 9% to 13%
Having first-degree relative with CD	5.5% to 9.5% (potentially 18% in siblings)

guidelines regarding screening. The guideline approach has broken screening into the following 2 groups:

1. Those with increased suspicion based on genetic predisposition

2. Those with increased suspicion based on signs and symptoms

The genetic predisposition group is summarized in Table 29-1 that provides the various associated conditions as well as estimated prevalence. Those with a genetic risk could be screened starting after 3 years of age (sooner if clinical concerns develop) and retested at regular— although not well defined—intervals, usually every 1 to 5 years. In their revised celiac guidelines, ESPGHAN is recommending human leukocyte antigen (HLA) testing as first-line screening for these at-risk genetic individuals. Negative HLA DQ2 and DQ8 results make the possibility of developing CD in an individual extremely unlikely and no further screening would then be recommended. While this approach seems valid based on the evidence and should certainly be considered, HLA typing may be associated with significant cost to the family and development of suspicious symptoms would likely result in an IgA tissue transglutaminase (tTG) antibody test, regardless of the HLA result.

Persistent signs or symptoms associated with CD are listed in Table 29-2. None of these signs or symptoms is specific for CD, and a small minority of those screened will end up having CD. These clinical manifestations are often grouped into gastrointestinal (GI) features that are classical or nonclassical, extraintestinal, and more recently, neuropsychiatric.

When to send the child who presents with recurrent abdominal pain for celiac screening is less clear. The presence of family history of celiac or other autoimmune diseases[4] may prompt earlier screening, as would the presence of other signs or symptoms. Isolated abdominal pain may be the only presenting complaint in a small minority of celiacs, so the decision to screen or not is best left up to the practitioners clinical judgment.

Table 29-2
Presenting Features of Celiac Disease

Classic	*Extraintestinal*	*Non-classic GI*	*Neuropsychiatric*
	Osteoporosis/osteopenia[a]		
Failure to thrive[a]	Dermatitis herpetiformis[a]	Constipation[a]	Chronic fatigue[a]
Chronic diarrhea[a]	Dental enamel defects[a]	Gastroesophageal reflux (GER)[b]	Epilepsy/cerebral calcifications[b]
Abdominal distention[a]	Anemia[a]		Migraines[b]
Muscle wasting[a]	Aphthous stomatitis[a]		Depression[b]
Anorexia[a]	Abnormal liver function tests[a]		Ataxia[a]
Nausea and vomiting[a]	Pubertal delay[a]		Anxiety[b]
Abdominal pain[a]	Short stature[a]		Peripheral neuropathy[a]
	Amenorrhea[a]		
	Infertility[b]		
	Recurrent fetal loss[b]		
	Arthritis[b]/arthralgias		
	Alopecia[b]		
	Vitamin deficiencies[a]		

[a]Indicates prompt testing for CD should be done, usually with tTG, early in the evaluation. Other persistent signs or symptoms may lead to screening for CD at some point in the work-up (ie, constipation, vomiting, or reflux symptoms).
[b]Association less strong with celiac.

When to screen or rescreen at-risk individuals is controversial. At present, it is reasonable to begin screening genetically at-risk, asymptomatic individuals aged 3 years if gluten has been part of the diet. Negative testing does not rule out future development of CD, and so periodic retesting at selected intervals is advised (with varying recommendations from 1 to 3 years). Development of persistent signs or symptoms should prompt testing, even in the first year of life, if gluten has been present in the diet. Some data suggest that tTG may be less sensitive in those under 2 years of age and advocate use of endomysial antibody. Our experience has been that this is not necessary and tTG as the single test is sufficient.

References

1. Hoffenberg EJ. Should all children be screened for celiac disease? *Gastroenterology.* 2005;128(4 suppl 1):S98-S103.
2. Hill ID, Dirks MH, Liptak GS, et al. North American Society for Pediatric Gastroenterology, Hepatology, and Nutrition. Guideline for the diagnosis and treatment of celiac disease in children: recommendations of the North American Society for Pediatric Gastroenterology, Hepatology, and Nutrition. *J Pediatr Gastroenterol Nutr.* 2005;40(1):1-19.
3. Husby S, Koletzko S, Korponay-Szabo IR, et al; ESPGHAN Gastroenterology Committee, European Society for Pediatric Gastroenterology, Hepatology, and Nuturition. The European Society for Pediatric Gastroenterology, Hepatology, and Nuturition guidelines for the diagnosis of coeliac disease diagnosis [published erratum appears in *J Pediatr Gastroenterol Nutr.* 2012;54(4):572]. *J Pediatr Gastroenterol Nutr.* 2012;54(1):136-160.
4. Sattar N, Lazare F, Kacer M, et al. Celiac disease in children, adolescents, and young adults with autoimmune thyroid disease. *J Pediatr.* 2011;158(2):272-275.

Review Articles

Bonamico M, Mariani P, Mazzilli MC, et al. Frequency and clinical pattern of celiac disease among siblings of celiac children. *JPGN.* 1996;23(2):159-163.
Van Koppen EJ, Schweizer JJ, Csizmadia CG, et al. Long-term health and quality-of-life consequences of mass screening for childhood celiac disease: a 10-year follow-up study. *Pediatrics.* 2009;123(4):e582-e588.

WHAT IS THE BEST WAY TO DIAGNOSE CELIAC DISEASE? WHAT IS THE ROLE OF HUMAN LEUKOCYTE ANTIGEN TYPING, SEROLOGY, AND SMALL INTESTINAL BIOPSY?

Alan M. Leichtner, MD and Dascha C. Weir, MD

Celiac disease (CD) is an immune-mediated enteropathy triggered by a permanent sensitivity to gluten, a term used to describe certain proteins in wheat, rye, and barley. It occurs in genetically susceptible individuals with a prevalence of approximately 1% of people in the United States and Europe and is being increasingly recognized in many other parts of the world. Children with autoimmune diseases (such as diabetes mellitus and thyroid disease), with genetic conditions (such as Down's syndrome or Turner's syndrome), or with a family history of CD are at higher risk of themselves having CD. Although it occurs commonly in pediatrics, CD has a wide and varied range of presentation in children and, therefore, can be easily overlooked.

The first step in making an accurate diagnosis of CD in children is recognizing when to look for it. The classic presentation of CD in patients in the toddler and preschool years is characterized by a syndrome of diarrhea, marked abdominal distention, abdominal pain, irritability, and failure to thrive. However, children with CD are now more often diagnosed in the elementary school years, at an average age of 9 years, and frequently have "atypical" symptoms. Some children who are tested because of associated diseases or a family history are completely asymptomatic.[1]

Gastrointestinal symptoms in children with CD include recurrent abdominal pain, nausea, vomiting, diarrhea, constipation, abdominal distention, increased gassiness, and decreased appetite. In our experience, constipation is seen as frequently as diarrhea as a presenting symptom. Common extraintestinal symptoms include weight loss or poor weight gain, short stature, pubertal delay, and fatigue. However, we also see children who are overweight or even obese at the time of presentation. It is important to recognize that children can also present in a myriad of other ways, including iron deficiency anemia, oral ulcers, arthritis, behavioral problems, dental enamel defects, transaminase or pancreatic enzyme elevations, osteopenia, headaches, depression, seizures, ataxia, hypotonia, and neuropathy. Children may have many, one, or none of these signs and symptoms.[2]

When your level of suspicion about CD is raised, either because of a child's clinical presentation, another high risk diagnosis, or a family history of CD, the next step is to order appropriate

Table 30-1
Test Performance of Celiac Serologic Markers

Antibody test	Sensitivity	Specificity
tTG (IgA)	●●●●	●●●◕
Endomysial (IgA)	●●●◕	●●●●
Gliadin (IgA and IgG)	●	●
Deamidated gliadin (IgA and IgG)	●●●●	●●●◕

celiac serology. We do not recommend sending a celiac panel as many of the tests included are unnecessary and expensive. The IgA (Immunoglobulin A) anti-tissue transglutaminase antibody (tTG), usually assayed by enzyme-linked immunosorbent assay, is the best test to send as it is highly sensitive, specific, and readily available (Table 30-1). It is important to send a total IgA-level at the same time as selective-IgA deficiency is more common in patients with CD, and these patients may not be able to mount a positive-IgA titer. IgG-based celiac serology is available, but these tests do not perform as well as IgA-based serology. If a child is deemed at risk of having CD and has concurrent IgA deficiency, we typically proceed to small bowel biopsy for further evaluation and forgo ordering IgG-based serology.

IgA anti-endomysial antibodies are another good marker with high specificity for CD, but this test is more technically difficult, more operator dependent, and usually more expensive than IgA-tTG. IgA and IgG anti-gliadin antibodies are less sensitive and specific tests that have been used in the recent past in patients under 2 years of age when other celiac serology may not be positive. A new test for antibodies to deamidated gliadin peptide is now available and may prove to be promising in pediatrics, but current studies suggest that it is fairly equivalent to IgA-tTG at this time.[3] IgG anti-deamidated gliadin peptide antibodies may be helpful in cases of IgA deficiency. If IgA-tTG testing is negative, but there is a high concern for CD in a patient in whom endoscopy is considered high risk, ordering additional serologic markers, such as the IgA anti-endomysial antibody or deamidated gliadin peptide antibodies, may be helpful.

Serologic testing, though helpful in determining who needs additional evaluation as well as supportive in making the diagnosis of CD, is not definitive. Approximately 10% of patients with biopsy-proven CD have negative serology. Conversely, some patients with positive serology do not have active CD on the small bowel biopsy. Therefore, positive serology alone is not enough to make the diagnosis of CD and a gluten-free diet should not be initiated without biopsy confirmation. Some pediatric gastroenterologists feel that children with very high titers of IgA-tTG, clinical signs and symptoms that are consistent with CD, and high risk for CD do not need confirmatory biopsies. Regardless, we recommend that all patients with positive celiac serology and all patients with negative serology but a high clinical suspicion for CD be referred to a pediatric gastroenterologist for additional evaluation.

Genetic testing, specifically human leukocyte antigen typing, can be helpful in some cases. While virtually all patients with CD test positive for DQ2 or DQ8, approximately 25% of patients in the general population have either DQ2 or DQ8 and clearly not all of these people develop CD. In our experience, this expensive testing is only helpful if neither haplotype is found. CD in a DQ2-negative and DQ8-negative person is exceedingly unlikely, though not impossible.[4] Nonetheless, in most cases, it is our current practice to proceed as if patients with negative celiac HLA typing do not have CD.

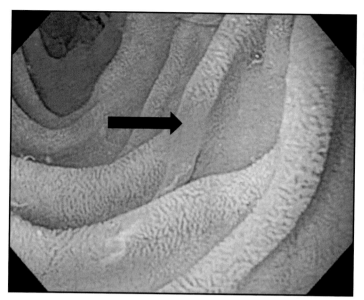

Figure 30-1. High-resolution endoscopic image of the duodenum demonstrating patchy villous atrophy (arrow). (Reprinted with permission from Dr. Victor Fox, Children's Hospital Boston, MA.)

The current gold standard for the diagnosis of CD remains the histopathologic examination of biopsies of the small intestine obtained by esophagogastroduodenoscopy. In pediatric patients, this procedure is done with general anesthesia, or sedation in cooperative, older children. Grossly evident small bowel changes, such as flattening of villi, scalloped folds, and other signs of inflammation, may be noted during endoscopy, but accurate diagnosis is based on examination of duodenal biopsies. In pediatric CD, duodenal biopsies are remarkable for villous blunting, crypt hyperplasia, and increased intraepithelial lymphocytes that are graded by the Marsh criteria. The biopsy findings characteristic of CD may be patchy in distribution (Figure 30-1) and may be noted only in the duodenal bulb.[5] Therefore, our standard practice is to ensure adequate sampling with at least 2 duodenal bulb biopsies and 4 biopsies in the more distal duodenum. If all biopsies are negative, but a high concern for CD remains, wireless capsule endoscopy, which permits visualization of the mucosa of the entire small intestine, may demonstrate villous atrophy consistent with CD.

Treatment with a gluten-free diet is indicated once the diagnosis of CD is confirmed, but not before. Both serologic testing and small bowel biopsy must occur while the child is ingesting gluten for a minimum of 4 to 6 weeks and ideally longer to assure accuracy of diagnosis. Also, since the gluten-free diet is restrictive and expensive, it is important to get the diagnosis right and make sure a child has CD before starting the diet.

References

1. Telega G, Bennet TR, Werlin S. Emerging new clinical patterns in the presentation of celiac disease. *Arch Pediatr Adolesc Med.* 2008;162(2):164-168.
2. Zawahir S, Safta A, Fasano A. Pediatric celiac disease. *Curr Opin Pediatr.* 2009;21(5):655-660.
3. Agardh D. Antibodies against synthetic deamidated gliadin peptides and tissue transglutaminase for the identification of childhood celiac disease. *Clin Gastroenterol Hepatol.* 2007;5(11):1276-1281.
4. Sollid L, Lie BA. Celiac disease genetics: current concepts and practical applications. *Clin Gastroenterol Hepatol.* 2005;3(9):843-851.
5. Weir DC, Glickman JN, Roiff T, Valim C, Leichtner AM. Variability of histopathological changes in childhood celiac disease. *Am J Gastroenterol.* 2010;105(1):207-12. Epub 2009 Oct 6.

31

WHY HAVE FOOD ALLERGIES BECOME SO COMMON AND WHAT ARE THE MOST ACCURATE MEANS OF DIAGNOSIS?

Scott H. Sicherer, MD

Has the prevalence of food allergies truly increased or is there simply a more liberal diagnosis? Numerous studies using different methodologies now indicate an increase in prevalence of food allergies.[1] For example, peanut allergy appears to have tripled in prevalence in children in the United States from about 0.4% in 1997 to 1.4% in 2008. Remarkably, this increased rate matches recent studies in Canada, Australia, and the United Kingdom. Overall, 4% to 8% of children have food allergies. It is not likely that anaphylactic reactions were simply missed decades ago, and there is also evidence of increases in other allergic diseases such as asthma, allergic rhinitis (hay fever), and atopic dermatitis (eczema); therefore, this increase appears to be quite real.

As for why there is an increase, there are a number of hypotheses. Leading the list of theories is the hygiene hypothesis, which suggests that our immune system is dysregulated because it is not sufficiently challenged by common pathogens. With numerous vaccinations, less farm living, smaller family sizes, and rampant use of antibiotics, this theory seems cogent. The immune system is looking for an enemy and mistakenly attacks foods. However, many other possibilities exist, including changes in how foods are processed that may increase allergenicity, increased obesity resulting in an inflammatory state, vitamin D deficiency causing immune dysregulation, and chemicals in the environment. Timing of the introduction of foods has also been scrutinized. Past suggestions about avoiding allergenic foods, such as eggs and peanuts, until well past the first year of life in families with allergy risk factors have been rescinded in favor of a less regimented approach and a liberalized diet, unless there are already signs of allergic disease.[2]

Despite the increased rate of food allergies, many families, perhaps 15% to 30%, avoid foods under an assumption of allergies.[1] Therefore, as the pediatrician, you are faced with a large number of children who require a careful approach to diagnosis that, thankfully, is likely to liberalize their diet.

The most important test toward an accurate diagnosis is the medical history. The history is used to determine whether a food-related disease is likely due to immune responses (allergy) or other adverse reactions, such as intolerance (eg, lactose intolerance), toxins (food poisoning), or pharmacologic responses (eg, caffeine). Details about symptoms, timing with meals, and the foods involved should allow a distinction among these causes of adverse reactions to foods and identify potential culprit foods.

When it comes time for laboratory tests, you do not want to pick the wrong test or misinterpret the results. Therefore, it is important to understand the distinctions among food allergies that are IgE (Immunoglobulin E) antibody-mediated, for which tests are available, and those that are not IgE antibody-mediated where simple tests are not available. IgE antibody-mediated food allergies include acute reactions within minutes, such as urticaria, vomiting, wheezing, or anaphylaxis. However, food allergies can also be caused by cellular responses, and these disorders are not associated with positive tests for IgE antibodies to foods. Examples include gastrointestinal (GI) reactions, such as proctocolitis and food protein-induced enterocolitis syndrome. Finally, there are disorders that are both cell-mediated and IgE-mediated, such as atopic dermatitis and eosinophilic esophagitis, where available tests are of limited value. Decisions about testing depend heavily upon distinguishing the pathohysiology of the reactions because tests for IgE antibodies may not have relevance to cell-mediated food allergies.

An accurate diagnosis is aided by understanding the epidemiology of food allergies. Most reactions are attributed to milk, egg, wheat, soy, peanut, tree nuts (eg, walnuts and cashews), fish, and shellfish. Allergies to milk, egg, wheat, and soy typically resolve in childhood while allergies to peanuts, nuts, fish, and shellfish are typically long-lived. When a child has a reaction, it is not only more likely due to one of these foods, but it is also more likely due to a food that is not already a frequently tolerated component of the child's current diet. For a child with a known food allergy, a new reaction might be caused by an accidental exposure to a known problem food rather than a new allergy.

Once the history identifies a type of adverse reaction and its relationship to food, the pathophysiology should be considered and triggers identified for appropriate test selection. Recommendations about diagnosis were recently published by an expert panel convened by the National Institute of Allergy and Infectious Diseases (NIAID) of the National Institute of Health (NIH), whose recommendations were based upon an extensive literature review.[3] The major recommendations are underscored by the notion that a food-allergy diagnosis cannot be easily achieved by simple tests (blood or skin tests), but rather, require consideration of the history.

The most commonly available laboratory allergy test is the serum test for food-specific IgE. This test, like the skin-prick test performed by allergists, is able to detect a sensitized state where the body is producing IgE antibodies that can recognize at least one and perhaps several proteins in the food tested. However, it is entirely possible for a test to be positive but the food is tolerated. About 8% of the United States population has a positive test to peanut, but almost all of these persons are tolerating peanut. Therefore, these tests are simply a guide. The higher the level of food-specific IgE, the more likely there is a true allergy. Because it is possible to be sensitized but not allergic, it is important to avoid ordering tests to foods that are already tolerated in the child's diet. Testing should be focused on possible culprits. It becomes difficult for you to explain a positive test to a food that was not causing any trouble, so be careful about ordering large panels of food tests.

Several tests are not recommended because they were shown to have no clinical value or remain unproven, including food-IgG/IgG4, applied kinesiology (muscle strength testing), provocation neutralization, hair analysis, and electrodermal testing.

There are additional test limitations and caveats for food-specific IgE testing. Sometimes the test is negative despite a true allergy. This may happen because the specific protein that is problematic to the patient is not well represented in the test. Therefore, trust your history and instincts and do not recommend that a child retry a food when the test is negative but the history is compelling. In this case, referral to an allergist for additional testing is warranted.

Another example where a negative test may be misleading is when the illness is not IgE-mediated. A good example is food protein-induced enterocolitis syndrome. Infants or children with this disorder develop severe vomiting and diarrhea and may have failure to thrive, acidemia, thrombocytosis, and elevated white blood cell counts with neutrophilia and bandemia. However, this disorder is not associated with food-specific IgE. Tests will be negative. The diagnosis is based upon classical history, which may include a 2-hour period between ingestion and symptom onset, and evaluations may include supervised feeding tests.

In fact, allergy confirmation for any type of food-allergic disorder often requires a medically supervised feeding test. This is the most accurate diagnostic test for food allergy. With this test, the clinician (typically an allergist) administers the food test gradually while evaluating for any symptoms. The gold standard format of this test is the double-blind, placebo-controlled oral-food challenge, where the test food is hidden and the feeding involves periods with placebo and true allergen administration to avoid biases.

However, allergy and feeding tests are not always sufficient. An example of a food-related GI disorder that requires a unique focused diagnostic routine is eosinophilic esophagitis.[4] Patients with this illness may have symptoms that mimic gastroesophageal reflux disease (GERD), but they are recalcitrant to reflux therapies and may also have symptoms of dysphagia or develop food impaction. A biopsy is required for diagnosis revealing significant esophageal eosinophilic inflammation despite aci-blockade therapy. Most children with this disorder will have food-responsive disease, but allergy test results do not correlate well with trigger foods. Therefore, testing is mostly ancillary to provide some guidance to empiric dietary trials that are followed by symptom response and rebiopsy. Medical management (ie, steroids) is also often required.

Once a diagnosis of food allergy is confirmed, education about food avoidance is key to prevent reactions. This includes information about label reading, cross-contact of allergens (unintended contamination during food preparation), and management in restaurants and school. Nutritional evaluation and growth monitoring of children with food allergy is recommended. Management of anaphylaxis requires prompt administration of epinephrine, and therefore self-injectors are prescribed for those with potentially life-threatening allergies. Management also requires education about when and how to use epinephrine autoinjectors, advice for observation for 4 to 6 hours or longer in an emergency department after treatment, and encouraging the child to wear medical identification jewelry. Consideration for consultation with an allergist-immunologist is advised. Educational materials are available through an NIH/NIAID sponsored consortium (www.cofar-group.org) and via websites of lay organizations (such as www.foodallergy.org and www.faiusa.org).

References

1. Sicherer SH. Epidemiology of food allergy. *J Allergy Clin Immunol.* 2011;127(3):594-602.
2. Greer FR, Sicherer SH, Burks AW, American Academy of Pediatrics Committee on Nutrition, American Academy of Pediatrics Section on Allergy and Immunology. Effects of early nutritional interventions on the development of atopic disease in infants and children: the role of maternal dietary restriction, breastfeeding, timing of introduction of complementary foods, and hydrolyzed formulas. *Pediatrics.* 2008;121(1):183-191.
3. Boyce JA, Assa'ad A, Burks AW, et al. NIAID-Sponsered Expert Panel. Guidelines for the diagnosis and management of food allergy in the United States: summary of the NIAID-Sponsored Expert Panel report. *J Allergy Clin Immunol.* 2010;126(6):1105-1118.
4. Liacouras CA, Furuta GT, Hirano I, et al. Eosinophilic esophagitis: updated consensus recommendations for children and adults. *J Allergy Clin Immunol.* 2011;128(1):3-20.

32

WHAT IS EOSINOPHILIC ESOPHAGITIS AND WHAT DO I DO ABOUT IT?

Shauna Schroeder, MD and Glenn T. Furuta, MD

Eosinophilic esophagitis (EoE) is defined as a chronic, immune-mediated esophageal disease characterized clinically by symptoms related to esophageal dysfunction and histologically by eosinophil-predominant inflammation. Following the trend of other allergic diseases, EoE is becoming recognized as an increasingly common cause of swallowing problems and reflux-like symptoms in children and adults.

What Clinical Features Are Suggestive of Eosinophilic Esophagitis?

EoE has a wide spectrum of presenting complaints that vary according to the age of presentation. Young children can present with commonplace symptoms, such as vomiting, abdominal pain, and feeding difficulties, that in some cases may lead to failure to thrive. Key historical features of feeding problems, such as food refusal, low-variety of intake, poor-acceptance of new foods, holding food in the mouth, spitting out food, and prolonged meal times, should raise an index of suspicion for EoE as a diagnostic possibility. Questions that address feeding-coping mechanisms include: Does your child eat slowly, take small bites, chew excessively, "chipmunk" or hide food in his or her cheeks, require drinking after each bite, or avoid specific foods with dense textures like meat or bread? As children become older and are more able to describe symptoms, more typical reflux-like symptoms such as heartburn, regurgitation, as well as dysphagia may be reported. Finally, older children and adolescents may present with any of the above symptoms as well as food "sticking" and impactions; in fact in some series, over half of patients presenting to emergency departments with food impactions have EoE.

Patients with an atopic history are another group in which we would suspect EoE. A number of studies have identified the association of EoE with a number of comorbid-allergic diseases like allergies, asthma, atopic dermatitis, and peripheral eosinophilia.

What Should I Do if I Suspect Eosinophilic Esophagitis?

If EoE is suspected, first we would rule out other common causes for symptoms. For instance, treatment of suspected gastroesophageal reflux disease (GERD) in a child with heartburn would be indicated as GERD is certainly more common than EoE. Anatomic etiologies (ie, malrotation and congenital strictures) should be ruled out with an upper gastrointestinal series. When indicated by other symptoms, alternative causes of esophageal eosinophilia, such as infection (*Helicobacter pylori*), Crohn's disease, celiac disease, and hypereosinophilic syndrome, need to be addressed. Your early referrals to pediatric gastroenterologists can be helpful for further diagnostic evaluation if the cause of symptoms is not apparent.

To date, no diagnostic biomarkers for EoE exist. As such, systemic inflammatory laboratory tests such as C-reactive protein and erythrocyte sedimentation rate have not been useful in making an EoE diagnosis. While some patients may have peripheral eosinophilia and elevated serum IgE levels, it is difficult to know whether these are increased because of EoE or concomitant atopic diseases.

What Should I Expect From My Consultants?

Pediatric gastroenterologists play an important role in the care of patients suspected of having EoE. These subspecialists will evaluate your patient to make sure that no other conditions may be causing the presenting symptoms and if indicated, will perform an upper endoscopy to assess the esophageal mucosa with pinch biopsies. Biopsy samples containing more than 15 eosinophils provide histological confirmation of the diagnosis of EoE (Figure 32-1) as long as other causes for eosinophilia are excluded. Frequently, gastroenterologists will oversee therapeutic plans that can include dietary restrictions or topical steroid treatments. Lastly, gastroenterologists will follow up with patients to assess for any complications (eg, esophageal strictures, feeding difficulties, and food impactions) related to EoE.

The role of the allergist in the evaluation of a child with EoE continues to undergo definition. As food allergens likely play a significant role in EoE, a thorough evaluation for potential food allergies is indicated. If sensitization is identified with a radioallergosorbent test or a skin test, decisions will need to be made as to potential roles of identified foods in the pathogenesis of the esophageal inflammation; these specific foods are then removed from the diet. Important roles for the allergist are also to perform evaluations for and treatment of other atopic diseases to assist in caring for the overall atopic features often seen in children with EoE.

What Treatments Are Used to Care for Patients With Eosinophilic Esophagitis?

Therapeutic decision making can be guided by gastroenterologists, allergists, and in some cases both. The overall goal of treatment is to promote normal growth and development. Effective

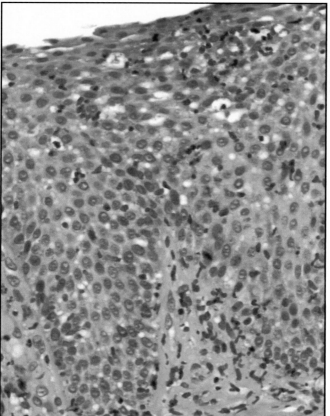

Figure 32-1. Esophageal biopsy with active esophagitis and inflammation characterized by marked basal zone hyperplasia, rete peg elongation, and infiltration of large numbers of eosinophils >15 eosinophils/high-power field (eos/hpf) (20x field of view).

treatments for EoE that resolve symptoms and resolve esophageal eosinophilia in the majority of patients include pharmacologic therapy with steroids and dietary management. The administration of steroids to the esophageal lining has been accomplished by using steroid preparations developed for the treatment of asthma. Metered-dose inhalers of fluticasone are directly sprayed in the mouth without inhaling or using a spacer with the intent that the saliva delivers medication to the esophageal lining. Alternatively, budesonide respules are mixed with sucralose to make a paste that when swallowed, provides a coating to the esophageal lining. Patients should not eat or drink for at least 30 minutes after taking the medication to maximize the contact time of the medication with the affected mucosa. While oral or esophageal *Candida* infections may be seen in some patients, systemic toxicities are rare. Systemic corticosteroids may be used in acute, emergent cases when patients have severe dysphagia requiring hospitalization because of weight loss and dehydration.

    Nutritional management of EoE is based on removal of offending allergens and can include the sole use of elemental formula, removal of potential food allergens based on allergy testing, or the empiric elimination of the 8 most common food-allergen groups: milk, soy, egg, wheat, shellfish, fish, tree nuts, and peanuts. The use of this approach should be undertaken with the guidance of a dietician to insure that the resulting diet is nutritionally replete.

References

1. Liacouras CA, Furuta GT, Hirano I, et al. Eosinophilic esophagitis: updated consensus recommendations for children and adults. *J Allergy Clin Immunol*. 2011;128(1):3-20.
2. Mukkada VA, Haas A, Maune NC, et al. Feeding dysfunction in children with eosinophilic gastrointestinal diseases. *Pediatrics*. 2010;126(3):e672-e677.
3. Schroeder S, Atkins D, Furuta GT. Recent advances in the treatment of eosinophilic esophagitis. *Expert Rev Clin Immunol*. 2010;6(6):929-937.

My Preteenaged Patient Has Chronic, Recurrent Epigastric Pain and a Blood Test Showed Immunoglobulin-G Antibodies Against Helicobacter pylori. Should I Start Helicobacter pylori-Eradication Therapy or Am I Missing Something?

Benjamin D. Gold, MD, FAAP, FACG

Abdominal pain is a frequent complaint of school-aged patients where up to 40% of children 4- to 18-years-old will have recurrent, nonlocalizable abdominal pain up to 3 times per week, randomly, and without any definitive etiology at some point in time in their lives.[1-3] Abdominal complaints like pain, nausea, or other dyspeptic symptoms are nonspecific and can be caused by different organic diseases within and outside the digestive tract. These diseases may be missed, or their diagnosis and treatment delayed, if a noninvasive test for *Helicobacter pylori* (*H pylori*) infection is positive and treatment initiated. In addition and more importantly, deciding the right time to test for *H pylori* infection and what specific tests to use poses a clinical dilemma for both the pediatrician in clinical practice and/or to the subspecialist pediatric gastroenterologist. The diagnostic dilemma for both the general pediatrician and consulting pediatric gastroenterologists can be further confused if the diagnostic test chosen, or inadvertently used, is a serological test (ie, blood test) that detects circulating antibodies against *H pylori* antigens (eg, immunoglobulin-G [IgG]). In each evidence-based clinical practice guideline for the management of pediatric *H pylori* infection published, it has been clear and without controversy, that commercially-available serology testing for antibodies specific for *H pylori* in the clinical setting are not recommended for use in the pediatric patient. Yet, clinicians continue to use serology as part of the initial approach to the diagnosis of *H pylori* infection—and more often than not—do not know how to deal with the results revealed by these highly inaccurate tests.[4]

H pylori demonstrates declining prevalence in developed countries and yet is one of the most common human infections world wide. To date, the primary period of *H pylori* acquisition is early childhood via fecal-oral, oral-oral, and gastro-oral mechanisms and no nonhuman reservoirs have been definitively identified. *H pylori* infection causes gastritis, duodenal and gastric ulcers, as well as gastric adenocarcinoma and mucosal-associated lymphoid type (MALT) lymphoma. More recently, *H pylori* has also been associated with extra-gastric conditions including growth failure, iron-deficiency anemia, and chronic idiopathic thrombocytopenia purpura. Ground-breaking investigations by El-Omar et al[5-6] showed that bacterial virulence, host-factors, and potentially environmental exposures play a role in the type of gastroduodenal inflammation and in disease outcome associated with *H pylori* disease.

The Pathogen and Its Epidemiology

H pylori is a gram-negative, motile, spiral-shaped bacillus that resides in a unique, biological niche: the human gastric mucosa. A number of *Helicobacter* species have been identified, with *H pylori* being the most common and the primary pathogen associated with human disease.[7-9] *H pylori* is a microaerophilic bacterium that devotes more than half of its energy producing significant quantities of the urease enzyme to successfully maintain persistence in the human stomach. *H pylori* resides in the stomachs of more than 50% of the world's population and the prevalence of this organism varies widely according to different geographic areas, age, race, and socioeconomic status. Despite overall decline in prevalence rates, childhood is the period in which most new *H pylori* infections are acquired, especially in developing countries.

In the United States, ethnic differences can be noted in the prevalence of *H pylori* infection. In African American and Hispanic populations, as well as immigrant populations, there is a 2- to 6-fold increased risk of being seropositive compared to White subjects of higher socioeconomic status. Overall, no gender differences are evident in the prevalence of *H pylori* infection but may play a role in the disease outcome. Poor hygiene in the living environment, particularly during childhood, correlate with higher prevalence. A number of studies have demonstrated that the socioeconomic status of the family in which the child is raised is inversely associated with *H pylori* prevalence.

Clinical Manifestations

H pylori infection in children generally results in a lack of clinically apparent symptoms. However, once there is persistent colonization, mucosal inflammation is almost universally associated. There are a number of reports of spontaneous elimination of *H pylori* infection in children. However, many of these studies are limited by the methodology used to determine infection presence/absence. Thus, it is not known how many children actually clear their infection spontaneously, and in the few cases reported, the underlying reasons are not known. Nodular gastritis appears to be a finding more consistently observed in children; however, the duration of time to develop these endoscopically-visible nodules and their natural history remains uncharacterized. In addition, which children with lympho-follicular gastritis progress to develop MALT lymphoma and over what time period remains another area for future research? Moreover, studies have demonstrated that eradication of *H pylori* in children with MALT lymphoma results in resolution of the mucosal disease, both gastric and extra gastric.

Although only case reports exist of gastric cancer development in children, early childhood acquisition of *H pylori* significantly increases the risk of this type of cancer. Moreover, our group and now others have demonstrated that atrophic gastritis and intestinal metaplasia, precursor

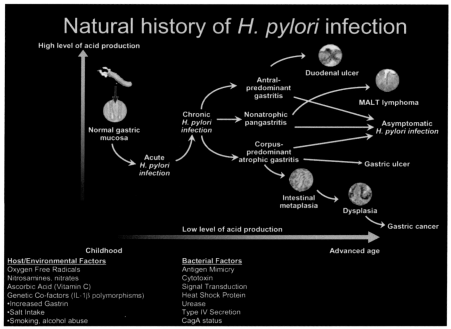

Figure 33-1. Pathogenesis and natural history of *H pylori* following initial ingestion. Determinants of disease outcome are bacterial, host, and environmental. (Adapted from Suerbaum S, Michetti P. *Helicobacter pylori* infection. *N Engl J Med.* 2002;347[15]:1175-1186.)

lesions for gastric cancer, occur in children infected by *H pylori*. These authors also showed that relatives of cancer patients had a higher prevalence of atrophy (34%) than patients with nonnuclear dyspepsia (5%) matched for *H pylori* prevalence. Thus, relatives of patients with gastric cancer have an increased prevalence of precancerous gastric abnormalities, but this increase is confined to those with *H pylori* infection. Because of these findings, pediatric guidelines have been changed to reflect a prophylactic eradication or prevention strategy in selected patients.

The natural history of *H pylori* infection appears to occur in phases (Figure 33-1). In studies of adult volunteers, an initial phase of intense-bacterial proliferation with gastric inflammation is observed and may briefly be associated with upper gastrointestinal (GI) symptoms and hypochlorhydria. How the natural history phases of infection relate to *H pylori* acquisition in either high- or low-endemic regions remains unclear. A chronic phase follows in which the inflammatory response is reduced to either a chronic diffuse superficial gastritis with normal and/or increased gastric pH, or antral predominant gastritis resulting in increased gastric-acid output and higher predilection for ulcer disease. Why the chronically infected person may remain free of symptoms for years or even a lifetime remains unclear.

To date, a causal relationship between *H pylori* infection and recurrent abdominal pain of childhood has not been definitively established. In addition, there seems to be a relationship between ulcer disease and abdominal symptoms, but it is still unclear whether chronic gastritis causes symptoms in children. Results from studies around the world have been conflicting and a definitive statement regarding treatment of *H pylori* found in the child with GI symptoms but no demonstrable disease remains a point of contention.

Further, *H pylori* infection in children does not appear to cause any specific symptoms. Epigastric pain, abdominal pain causing nocturnal wakening, hematemesis, and recurrent vomiting are not predictive of *H pylori* infection as no difference has been found between colonized and noncolonized children.

Diagnosis

At present, there are no specific symptoms or constellation of signs and symptoms that can predict the presence of gastritis or peptic ulcers in children. Furthermore, the majority of *H pylori* infection and the associated gastritis generally remain asymptomatic. However, children with warning symptoms or alarm signs, such as severe, chronic abdominal pain, anorexia, failure to thrive, or persistent vomiting, require investigation. The presence of occult blood in feces, particularly in the face of iron deficiency and/or iron-deficiency anemia should be investigated first. The severity of symptoms determines the need for endoscopy and with respect to *H pylori*, endoscopy and biopsy is done to determine the cause of symptoms, not just the infection.

As per the most recently published, comprehensive North American Society for Pediatric Gastroenterology, Hepatology, and Nutrition (NASPGHAN) and European Society for Pediatric Gastroenterology, Hepatology, and Nutrition (ESPGHAN) guidelines, the following 4 questions were addressed using the methodology described:

1. Who should be tested? (ie, differentiating among screening, surveillance, and clinically-based screening)
2. What tests should be used?
3. Who should be treated?
4. What treatment regimens are the most appropriate?

The recommendations for diagnostic testing include the following:

- The primary goal of clinical investigation of GI symptoms is to determine the underlying cause of the symptoms and not solely the presence of *H pylori* infection.

- Diagnostic testing for *H pylori* infection is not recommended in children with functional abdominal pain.

- In children with first-degree relatives with gastric cancer, testing for *H pylori* may be considered.

- In children with refractory iron-deficiency anemia, in which other causes have been ruled out, testing for *H pylori* infection may be considered (this recommendation being something new that had not been previously recommended for diagnostic testing in other published guidelines).

- For the diagnosis of *H pylori* infection during esophagogastroduodenoscopy, it is recommended that gastric biopsies (antrum and corpus) for histopathology are obtained.

- It is recommended that the initial diagnosis of *H pylori* infection be based on either a positive histopathology plus a positive rapid-urease test, or a positive culture.

- The 13C-urea breath test (UBT) is a reliable noninvasive test to determine whether *H pylori* has been eradicated.

- A validated enzyme-linked immunosorbent assay (ELISA) test for detection of *H pylori* antigen in stool is a reliable noninvasive test to determine whether *H pylori* has been eradicated.

- Tests based on the detection of antibodies (IgG, IgA) against *H pylori* in serum, whole blood, urine, and saliva are not reliable for use in the clinical setting.

- It is recommended that clinicians wait at least 2 weeks after stopping proton pump inhibitor (PPI) therapy and 4 weeks after stopping antibiotics to perform biopsy-based and noninvasive tests (UBT, stool test) for *H pylori*.

Treatment

According to the evidence-based NASPGHAN and ESPGHAN clinical practice guidelines for the management of pediatric *H pylori* infection, treatment is indicated in the following clinical scenarios:

1. In the presence of *H pylori*-positive peptic ulcer disease (PUD), eradication of the organism is recommended.

2. When *H pylori* infection is detected by biopsy-based methods in the absence of PUD, *H pylori* treatment is recommended.

3. A test-and-treat strategy is not recommended in children.

4. In children who are infected with *H pylori* and whose first-degree relative has gastric cancer, treatment may be offered.

5. First-line eradication regimens include the following:

   ○ Triple therapy with a PPI + amoxicillin + clarithromycin

   ○ An imidazole bismuth salts + amoxicillin + an imidazole

   ○ Sequential therapy

6. It is recommended that the duration of triple-therapy be 7 to 14 days.

Cost, compliance, and adverse effects should be taken into account. Additionally, both the updated Canadian recommendations and the recently published NASPGHAN and ESPGHAN guidelines include treatment for symptomatic infection in a child with a family history of gastric cancer, and make strong suggestions to screen and treat an infected child with a family history of gastric cancer and asymptomatic.

Of the 2 updated pediatric guidelines, the more recent NASPGHAN and ESPGHAN guidelines provide an algorithm to assist the clinician in the decision-making process when evaluating a child with suspected *H pylori* (Figure 33-2). The most effective anti-*Helicobacter* therapy currently accepted for children is a 2-week triple-therapy that includes a PPI, such as omeprazole (1 mg/kg/day) or lansoprazole, along with clarithromycin (15 mg/kg/day) and amoxicillin (50 mg/kg/day). Table 33-1 depicts a list of the accepted, evidence-based, and most effective eradication therapies for children.

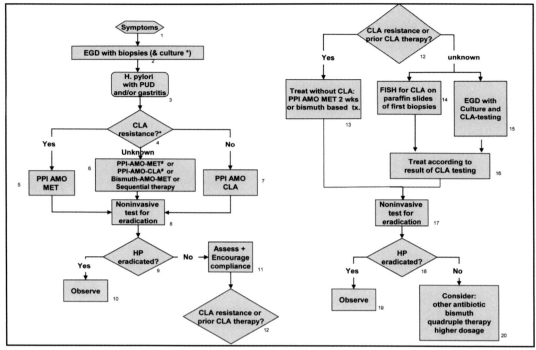

Figure 33-2. Proposed algorithm to treat *H. pylori* infection in pediatric patients. EGD: esophagogastro-duodenoscopy; PUD: peptic ulcer disease; CLA: clarithromycin. *In areas or populations with a primary clarithromycin resistance rate of >20% or unknown background antibiotic resistance rates, culture and susceptibility testing should be performed and treatment should be chosen accordingly. #If susceptibility testing has not been performed or has failed, antibiotics should be chosen according to the background of the child. (Reprinted with permission from Koletzko S, Jones NL, Goodman KJ, et al. Evidence-based guidelines from ESPGHAN and NASPGHAN for Helicobacter pylori infection in children. *J Pediatr Gastroenterol Nutr.* 2011;53(2):230-243.)

Table 33-1
First-Line Treatment Recommendations for *Helicobacter pylori* Eradication in Children

- PPI (1 to 2 mg/kg/day)+amoxicillin (50 mg/kg/day)+metronidazole (20 mg/kg/day)[a]
- PPI (1 to 2 mg/kg/day)+amoxicillin (50 mg/kg/day)+clarithromycin (20 mg/kg/day)[a]
- Bismuth salts (bismuth subsalicylate or subcitrate 8 mg/kg /day)+amoxicillin (50 mg/kg/day)+metronidazole (20 mg/kg/day)[a]
- PPI (1 to 2 mg/kg/day)+amoxicillin (50 mg/kg/day) for 5 days then PPI (1 to 2 mg/kg/day)+clarithromycin (20 mg/kg/day)+metronidazole (20 mg/kg/day) for 5 days

[a]Administered twice-daily for 10 to 14 days.
Note: PPI: proton pump inhibitor. Maximum daily dose is 2000 mg for amoxicillin, 1000 mg for metronidazole, 1000 mg/d for clarithromycin. (Reprinted with permission from Koletzko S, Jones NL, Goodman KJ, et al. Evidence-based guidelines from ESPGHAN and NASPGHAN for Helicobacter pylori infection in children. *J Pediatr Gastroenterol Nutr.* 2011;53(2):230-243.)

References

1. Sabbi T, Dall'Oglio L, De Angelis P, et al. Utility of a stool antigen test to detect the incidence of *helicobacter pylori* infection and familial and community environmental risk factors for this infection in pediatric age. *Pediatr Med Chir.* 2012;34(2):89-95.

2. Alfven G. Recurrent pain, stress, tender points and fibromyalgia in childhood: an exploratory descriptive clinical study. *Acta Paediatr.* 2012;101(3):283-291.

3. Ashorn M, Rago T, Kokkonen J, Ruuska T, Rautelin H, Karikoski R. Symptomatic response to *Helicobacter pylori* eradication in children with recurrent abdominal pain: double blind randomized placebo-controlled trial. *J Clin Gastroenterol.* 2004;38(8):646-650.

4. Chang HY, Sharma VK, Howden CW, Gold BD. Knowledge, attitudes, and practice styles of North American pediatric gastroenterologists: *Helicobacter pylori* infection. *J Pediatr Gastroenterol Nutr.* 2003;36(2):235-240.

5. El-Omar EM, Carrington M, Chow WH, et al. Interleukin-1 polymorphisms associated with increased risk of gastric cancer [published erratum Nature. 2001;412(6842):99]. *Nature.* 2000;404(6776):398-402.

6. El-Omar EM, Chow WH, Rabkin CS. Gastric cancer and *H pylori*: host genetics open the way. *Gastroenterology.* 2001;121(4):1002-1004.

7. Haesebrouck F, Pasmans F, Flahou B, Smet A, Vandamme P, Ducatelle R. Non-Helicobacter pylori *Helicobacter* species in the human gastric mucosa: a proposal to introduce the terms *H. heilmannii* sensu lato and sensu stricto. *Helicobacter.* 2011;16(4):339-340.

8. Nilsson HO, Pietroiusti A, Gabrielli M, Zocco MA, Gasbarrini G, Gasbarrini A. *Helicobacter pylori* and extragastric diseases–other *Helicobacters. Helicobacter.* 2005;10 suppl 1:54-65.

9. On SL. Taxonomy of *Campylobacter, Arcobacter, Helicobacter* and related bacteria: current status, future prospects and immediate concerns. *Symp Ser Soc Appl Microbiol.* 2001;(30):1S-15S.

10. Koletzko S, Jones NL, Goodman KJ, et al. Evidence-based guidelines from ESPGHAN and NASPGHAN for Helicobacter pylori infection in children. *J Pediatr Gastroenterol Nutr.* 2011;53(2):230-243.

34

Is Gastroesophageal Reflux Disease Really Common in Children and Adolescents? What Are the Best Ways to Diagnose and Treat It?

Steven J. Czinn, MD, FAAP, FACG, AGAF; Samra S. Blanchard, MD; Anayansi Lasso-Pirot, MD; and Adam Paul, DO

Gastroesophageal reflux (GER) is the physiologic phenomenon of involuntary passage of gastric contents into the esophagus with or without vomiting or regurgitation. GER frequently occurs postprandially and is asymptomatic. Gastroesophageal reflux disease (GERD) occurs when the gastric material refluxed causes significant, pathological conditions, including failure to thrive, poor weight gain, and chronic respiratory disorders, such as aspiration pneumonia, esophageal inflammation, apnea, hematemesis, or apparent life-threatening events. GERD is caused by transient relaxation of the lower esophageal sphincter (LES), causing an intragastric pressure that equals or exceeds that of the LES, allowing contents to travel retrograde into the esophagus. These transient relaxations are pathologic in nature when they occur unrelated to swallowing, or are longer in duration than the normal relaxation caused by swallowing. Other factors that influence GERD severity include esophageal-clearance time, intra-abdominal pressure, gastric compliance, delayed gastric emptying, and the composition of the refluxate.

Approximately 70% to 85% of infants have regurgitation with feedings at 2 months of life, and by about 3 to 4 months of life, 41% are still spitting up most of their feedings. Encouragingly, GER occurs in less than 5% of infants by 13 to 14 months of age without intervention. Even in patients treated for GERD in infancy, only about 10% have persistent symptoms into childhood and adolescence. A number of factors contribute to the frequency of regurgitation in infants. A shorter esophagus, small capacity of the esophagus, and frequent recumbent posture make it more likely that refluxed material in the infant will fill the esophagus and pass into the pharynx.

Regurgitation and vomiting, frequently described by parents as spitting up, are the most common symptoms of infantile GER. These episodes, occurring in well-appearing infants with normal growth, are effortless and painless. These patients are the so-called "happy spitters." Physical exam and a detailed feeding history including amount, frequency, and type of feeding, position during and after feedings, burping, and behavior during feedings, is sufficient to diagnose uncomplicated infant GER. Forceful or projectile emesis and coughing, choking, or gagging with feedings are warning signs that GERD or other diagnoses may be present. Fussiness and unexplained crying are nonspecific signs associated with a multitude of conditions in infants. When coupled with back arching, these symptoms may be seen as an expression of heartburn or chest pain associated with a reflux episode. Although uncommon, Sandifer's syndrome is described as opisthotonic posturing and arching of the back, which are a signs specific to GERD. When presented with this scenario, it is important to rule out other neurological disorders, such as seizures, infantile spasm, and dystonia. Though the exact mechanism is unclear, it appears to be related to esophageal acid exposure, as Sandifer's improves with antireflux treatment.

Complicated GERD is evident when the infant is experiencing poor weight gain, excessive irritability, food refusal, anemia, iron deficiency, dysphagia, odynophagia, feeding problems, or respiratory symptoms. Older children typically have more adult-like symptoms when it pertains to GERD. Heartburn, chest discomfort, regurgitation of foods, and epigastric pain are common complaints for children and adolescents with GERD.

The diagnosis of GER is generally made by history and physical alone. There is no symptom in infants that is diagnostic of GERD, and parent-reported infant-GERD questionnaires have been found to be unreliable. In infants, severity and frequency of symptoms are not reliable predictors of the degree of esophagitis. Complicated GER, or lack of response to empiric treatment, are indications for further work-up in both infants, older children, and adolescents. Diagnostic modalities include radiographic studies, endoscopy with biopsies, and esophageal pH monitoring with esophageal impedance. An upper gastrointestinal (GI) series is of low-diagnostic use for establishing GERD, but it does aid in identification of anatomic abnormalities, such as esophageal strictures or webs, hiatal hernia, intestinal malrotation, or pyloric stenosis. If there is a concern for aspiration during feeding, a modified-barium swallow should be ordered. Esophageal pH monitoring and impedance is a safe and effective means of diagnosing acid and weakly acid reflux in children. Esophageal impedance monitoring may aid in diagnosis when nonacid reflux is present. Multichannel-intraluminal impedance detects reflux episodes based on changes in electrical current between 2 electrodes on the probe when a liquid bolus passes between them. Esophageal pH monitoring is most useful in correlating symptoms (or perception of symptoms) to the pH at the time of the episode. It is important to take into account feeding time, positioning, and medication administration when interpreting a pH monitor report; pH monitoring may also be useful in determining efficacy of reflux treatment in patients who do not respond. Biopsies taken during an esophagogastroduodenoscopy may be used to determine extent or severity of esophageal damage caused by reflux. Visible lesions, including erosions, ulcerations, strictures, and exudates can be associated with GERD. Histologically, basal cell hyperplasia, increased papillary length, edema, erosions, and ulcerations are signs of reflux esophagitis.

Treatment of children with uncomplicated reflux begins with reassurance and lifestyle changes. In infants, effective burping, feeding positioning, and holding an infant upright for 20 to 30 minutes following feeds may provide some relief from normal physiologic regurgitation. Parental education about normal physiologic reflux and providing reassurance that the infant will likely outgrow the reflux is typically sufficient. While formula thickening may not reduce measurable reflux, adding rice cereal, corn or potato starch, carob-bean gum, carob-seed flour, or sodium carboxymethylcellulose to formula may decrease the frequency of regurgitation. Thickening formula with too much rice cereal may lead to excessive weight gain or constipation. Infants with a cow's milk or soy protein allergy may have regurgitation that mimics GERD. Replacing standard milk protein-based formula with a hydrolyzed- or amino acid-based formula may provide significant relief in 2 to 4 weeks time. In the breastfeeding mother, dietary restriction of milk and soy-containing products from the maternal diet should be considered.

For older children, conservative therapy is similar to recommendations for adults. Small, frequent meals in favor of large meals, avoiding a supine position immediately after eating, weight loss if obese, and avoidance of caffeinated products, chocolate, spicy foods, and high-fat foods may lead to improvement of reflux symptoms.

Medications currently used to treat GERD in infants and children are gastric-acid buffering agents, mucosal-surface barriers, antisecretory agents and prokinetic agents. Histamine 2-receptor antagonists (H2RAs) decrease acid secretion by inhibiting histamine-2 receptors on gastric parietal cells. Medications in this class include cimetidine, famotidine, nizatidine, and the most commonly used ranitidine. Tachyphylaxis can develop in all H2RAs, resulting in a decrease in acid suppression, and therefore tolerance can be seen as early as 14 days after initiation of therapy. The required optimal dose of ranitidine for preterm infants is 0.5 mg/kg body weight twice daily, and for term infants 1.5 mg/kg body weight 3 times daily. The oral dose for infants older than 1 month varies between 4 to 10 mg/kg/day divided twice daily, and the intravenous dose is 2 to 4 mg/kg/day divided twice daily. The cimetidine oral dose in infants is 10 to 20 mg/kg/day divided 2 to 4 times a day. Famotidine oral dose is 0.5 mg/kg/day once daily for newborns, and twice daily in infants older than 3 months. All H2RAs require dosing adjustment in renal impairment and can cause irritability and abnormal liver-function tests. Proton pump inhibitors (PPIs) inhibit acid secretion by blocking the sodium-potassium adenosine triphosphatase part of the proton pump that performs the final-step in acid secretion. PPIs are more efficacious due to their ability to maintain the pH above 4.0 for longer periods of time, and their inhibition of meal-induced acid secretion that H2RAs do not. PPIs are well tolerated, but common side effects include headache, diarrhea, rash, nausea, and constipation. PPIs currently approved for use in children include omeprazole, lansoprazole, and esomeprazole for children older than 1 year, and pantoprazole for children older than 5 years. Although not approved in the pediatric age group, PPIs are commonly used for treating GERD in infants. Antacids are a class of medications that work by neutralizing gastric acid, and thus minimizing the exposure of gastric acid to esophagus during a reflux episode. These agents contain magnesium and aluminum hydroxide or calcium carbonate. Agents containing aluminum can lead to osteopenia, microcytic anemia, and neurotoxicity due to elevated aluminum levels. Prokinetic agents improve regurgitation via their effects on LES pressure, peristalsis and acid clearance, or decreasing gastric emptying time. Metoclopramide and erythromycin are 2 of the more commonly used prokinetics in pediatrics. Metoclopramide has cholinoimetic and serotonergic effects, and may have some benefit in the symptomatic treatment of GERD, but these must be weighed against the side effect profile. Adverse effects include irritability, drowsiness, and extrapyramidal reactions while taking metaclopramide. Erythromycin, a commonly used macrolide antibiotic, acts on motilin receptors and thereby selectively improves gastric emptying in infants and children. The optimal dose for treating GI motility is 1 to 3 mg/kg/dose. There is a risk of developing hypertrophic pyloric stenosis when using erythromycin in infants younger than 6 months. To date, there are no published studies in infants evaluating safety and efficacy of erythromycin in GERD.

Antireflux surgical therapy in children is limited to children who fail medical therapy or who have life-threatening complications of GERD. Those who qualify are patients with neurological impairment or chronic respiratory conditions, including recurrent aspiration pneumonias or repaired esophageal atresia. Fundoplication, the wrapping of the fundus around the LES, is commonly performed by the Nissen method. This procedure can be performed both as an open surgery or laparoscopically.

GER, although usually self-limited, is a common complaint in the pediatric population. Nonpharmacologic therapy is considered first-line in the treatment. These approaches can be taught in the primary care setting to patients, and a 2-week trial is currently recommended by both the North American Society for Pediatric Gastroenterology, Hepatology, and Nutrition and the European Society for Pediatric Gastroenterology, Hepatology, and Nutrition. For infants and children who do not respond, a trial of acid suppression is warranted. Further evaluation by a pediatric gastroenterologist can be beneficial in the setting of complicated- or intractable-GERD following initial therapies.

Bibliography

Campanozzi A, Boccia G, Pensabene L, et al. Prevalence and natural history of gastroesophageal reflux: pediatric prospective survey. *Pediatrics*. 2009;123(3):779-783.

Coletti RB, DiLorenzo C. Overview of pediatric gastroesophageal reflux disease and proton pump inhibitor therapy. *J Pediatr Gastroenterol Nutr*. 2003;37(suppl 1):S7-S11.

Sherman PM, Hassall E, Fagundes-Neto U. A global, evidence-based consensus on the definition of gastroesophageal reflux disease in the pediatric population. *Am J Gastroenterol*. 2009;104(5):1278-1295.

Tighe MP, Afazal NA, Bevan A, Beattie RM. Current pharmacological management of gastro-esophageal reflux in children: an evidence-based systematic review. *Paediatr Drugs*. 2009;11(3):185-202.

Vandenplas Y, Rudolph CD, Di Lorenzo C, et al; North American Society for Pediatric Gastroenterology Hepatology and Nutrition, European Society for Pediatric Gastroenterology Hepatology and Nutrition. Pediatric gastroesophageal reflux clinical practice guidelines: joint recommendations of the North American Society for Pediatric Gastroenterology, Hepatology, and Nutrition (NASPGHAN) and the European Society for Pediatric Gastroenterology, Hepatology, and Nutrition (ESPGHAN). *J Pediatr Gastroenterol Nutr*. 2009;49(4):498-547.

QUESTION 35

WHAT TESTING IS NEEDED TO MAKE THE CORRECT DIAGNOSIS IN CHILDREN AND ADOLESCENTS WITH RECURRENT ABDOMINAL PAIN?

Silvana Bonilla, MD and Miguel Saps, MD

Recurrent abdominal pain (RAP) is one of the most common pediatric problems encountered in clinical practice. It affects up to 25% of school-aged children and adolescents and accounts for a significant number of consultations in the primary care setting. RAP was first defined by the British pediatrician John Apley as the occurrence of abdominal pain severe enough to interfere with daily functioning that occurs at least once a month over 3 consecutive months. RAP encompasses both organic and nonorganic etiologies that may account for the child's symptoms. The vast majority of children and adolescents presenting with RAP have a functional gastrointestinal disorder (FGID). FGIDs are a group of conditions defined by the presence of chronic or persistent symptoms occurring in the absence of biochemical, structural, or anatomical abnormalities. The term *RAP* has fallen into disuse particularly with the introduction of the Rome criteria for the diagnosis of pediatric FGIDs.

The Rome criteria are symptom-based criteria that assist in the diagnosis of nonorganic etiologies (including those related to chronic abdominal pain). They allow us to make a positive diagnosis of a FGID. A positive diagnosis helps in providing reassurance to patients, families, and physicians, thus reducing the need of unnecessary diagnostic and therapeutic interventions. The original criteria were revised in 2006 to produce the Rome III criteria. There are 4 recognized FGIDs associated with chronic abdominal pain lasting for more than 2 months, including functional dyspepsia, characterized by upper gastrointestinal (GI) symptoms; irritable bowel syndrome (IBS), characterized by chronic abdominal pain in the setting of changes in the stool frequency and/or consistency; functional abdominal pain (FAP), characterized by pain without stool changes; and abdominal migraine, characterized by paroxysmal episodes of pain followed by pain-free intervals (Table 35-1). The diagnosis of the different combinations of symptoms that characterize each functional GI disorder is facilitated by a set of validated questions (Questionnaire of Pediatric Gastrointestinal Symptoms). The questionnaire is completed either by parents of a child younger than 10 years or by the child when older than 10 years.

Table 35-1
Rome III Criteria for the Diagnosis of Pediatric Functional Gastrointestinal Disorders

Functional Dyspepsia[a,b]
Persistent or recurrent pain or discomfort centered in the upper abdomen (above the umbilicus)
Not relieved by defecation or associated with the onset of a change in stool frequency or stool form (ie, not IBS)

Irritable Bowel Syndrome[a,b]
Abdominal discomfort (an uncomfortable sensation not described as pain) or pain associated with 2 or more of the following at least 25% of the time: • Improved with defecation   • Onset associated with a change in frequency of stool   • Onset associated with a change in form (appearance) of stool

Abdominal Migraine[a,c]
Paroxismal episodes of intense, acute periumbilical pain that last for 1 hour or more
Interval periods of usual health lasting weeks to months
The pain interferes with normal activities
The pain is associated with 2 or more of the following: • Anorexia   • Nausea   • Vomiting   • Headache   • Photophobia   • Pallor

Functional Abdominal Pain[a,b]
Episodic or continuous abdominal pain
Insufficient criteria for other FGIDs

[a]No evidence of an inflammatory, anatomic, metabolic, or neoplastic process that explains the subject's symptoms.
[b]Criteria fulfilled at least once per week for at least 2 months before diagnosis.
[c]Criteria fulfilled 2 or more times in the preceding 12 months.

The conditions included in the differential diagnosis of RAP are extensive (Table 35-2). Whether any tests are needed should be addressed on a case-by-case basis according to the information obtained during the consultation (comprehensive history and physical examination), as well as the physician and family level of comfort with the clinical diagnosis. In order to make an educated decision on the use of testing, it is important to acknowledge the absence of almost any

Table 35-2
Possible Etiologies of Chronic Abdominal Pain

Organic Etiologies	
GI	
Esophagitis	CD
Gastritis	Polyps
Duodenitis	Parasites
Peptic ulcer	Hernias
Eosinophilic gastroenteritis	Tumors
Malrotation	Foreign body
Cysts (duplication or mesenteric)	Intussusception
Carbohydrate intolerance	IBD
Hepatobiliary	
Chronic hepatitis	Choledochal cyst
Cholecystitis	Sphincter of Oddi dysfunction
Cholelithiasis	
Pancreatic	
Pancreatitis	Pseudocyst
Gynecologic	
Hematocolpos	Mittelschmertz
Endometriosis	Tumor
Metabolic	
Porphyria	Lead poisoning
Diabetes	
Musculoskeletal	
Trauma	Infection
Inflammation	Tumor
Respiratory	
Infection, tumor, or inflammation in the vicinity of the diaphragm	
Urinary	
Ureteropelvic junction obstruction	Hydronephrosis
Recurrent pyelonephritis	Nephrolithiasis
Recurrent cystitis	

(continued)

Table 35-2 (continued)
Possible Etiologies of Chronic Abdominal Pain

Hematologic	
Angioedema	Sickle cell disease
Collagen vascular disease	
Psychiatric	
Conversion reaction	
Functional Etiologies	
FGID	
Functional dyspepsia	IBS
Abdominal migraine	Functional abdominal pain

GI: gastrointestinal; CD: celiac disease; IBD: irritable bowel disease; FGID: functional gastrointestinal disorder; IBS: irritable bowel syndrome.

data to justify the use of most of the tests that are frequently indicated. A technical report from the American Academy of Pediatrics and the North American Society for Pediatric Gastroenterology, Hepatology, and Nutrition (NASPGHAN) found limited evidence to recommend the use of testing in the absence of alarm signs in children with abdominal pain. Alarm signs, or "red flags," have classically been associated with organic etiologies (Table 35-3). These signs are useful in clinical practice as a guide for potential diagnostic evaluation. Unfortunately, they are not perfect and we should always remember that some of them might even be present in patients with FGIDs. For example, nocturnal pain may be present in up to a third of children with FGIDs. Fever, mouth ulcers, hematochezia, and weight loss can also be present in some children with FGIDs (approximately 1/20 cases). However, the absence of these alarm signs on a patient meeting criteria for a FGID makes the latter diagnosis even more likely.

Most clinicians use screening tests for patients in whom a diagnosis of FGID is suspected. Frequently ordered tests include a complete blood cell count with differential, chemistry panel, serum aminotransferases, celiac serology, erythrocyte sedimentation rate, thyroid function tests, urinalysis, and stool studies for blood, ova, and parasites. Other testing that has been suggested includes lactose breath hydrogen testing for lactose intolerance but the correlation between diagnosis and symptoms is low. Ultrasound of the abdomen has also been advocated but was found to have a poor diagnostic yield. In some cases, ultrasound proved to be detrimental by adding anxiety to the patient and family and prompting unnecessary consultation. The use of esophagogastroduodenoscopy is an invasive and expensive procedure that frequently detects subtle and nonspecific abnormalities that rarely affect the management in a substantial way. Some investigators argue that performing the procedure in patients with FGIDs provides reassurance to the families about

Table 35-3
Signs and Symptoms Suggesting Organic Etiology

Presence of more than one symptom	Perianal disease
Pain away from the umbilicus	Dysuria, hematuria
Nocturnal pain	Joint pain
Persistent vomiting	Fever
Hematemesis	Elevated inflammatory markers (eg, ESR and CRP)
Involuntary weight loss	Elevated white blood cell count
Growth deceleration	Anemia
Blood in the stools	Hypoalbuminemia
Changes in bowel function	Family history of IBD and/or peptic ulcer disease

ESR: erythrocyte sedimentation rate; CRP: C-reactive protein; IBD: inflammatory bowel disease.

the diagnosis and possibly improve outcomes. However, based on a recent study, children who had a negative endoscopy have a similar prognosis than those who did not. It is important to remember that in a patient with a history and physical examination consistent with FGIDs and a negative work-up, we should refrain from ordering further testing since these tests will likely be negative.

Conclusion

We should not rely on diagnostic testing to make a diagnosis. In children presenting with symptoms of RAP, functional disorders are much more common than organic diseases. Screening tests in children with FGIDs rarely show any clinically relevant abnormalities that will result in changes of management. Therefore, negative testing is the norm and clinicians should limit their testing, as those are likely to be negative. A negative test should be used as an opportunity to reassure the parents that the diagnosis is that of an FGID and not as a first step in further testing. In our experience, testing of patients with RAP should be done in an individualized manner guided by the information gathered on the history and physical examination. If the patient meets Rome criteria for FGIDs, we either do not conduct testing or conduct limited testing unless there is presence of alarm features suggestive of an organic etiology. Only in this case would we consider further testing with upper endoscopy with biopsies and/or imaging studies.

Bibliography

Bonilla S, Deli Wang, Saps M. The prognostic value of obtaining a negative endoscopy in children with functional gastrointestinal disorders. *Clin Pediatr (Phila)*. 2011;50(5):396-401.

Dhroove G, Chogle A, Saps M. A million-dollar work-up for abdominal pain: is it worth it? *J Pediatr Gastroenterol Nutr*. 2010;51(5):579-583.

Di Lorenzo C, Colletti RB, Lehmann HP, et al; AAP Subcommittee; NASPGHAN Committee on Chronic Abdominal Pain. Chronic aabdominal pain in children: a technical report of the American Academy of Pediatrics and the North American Society for Pediatric Gastroenterology, Hepatology, and Nutrition. *J Pediatr Gastroenterol Nutr*. 2005;40(3):249-261.

Rasquin A, Di Lorenzo C, Forbes D, et al. Childhood functional gastrointestinal disorders: child/adolescent. *Gastroenterology*. 2006;130(5):1527-1537.

WHAT TREATMENTS ARE AVAILABLE FOR PEDIATRIC RECURRENT ABDOMINAL PAIN AND WHICH ONES ACTUALLY WORK?

Jonathan E. Teitelbaum, MD

There is little evidence-based guidance for the treatment of functional gastrointestinal disorders (FGIDs) in children. Thus, therapy is driven by adult studies or anecdotal experience. Within the pediatric population, an evidence-based approach would suggest that the only effective therapies are cognitive behavioral therapy and placebo.

It is helpful to categorize patients with FGIDs into recurrent abdominal pain (RAP), irritable bowel syndrome with diarrhea-predominant (IBS-D) or constipation-predominant symptoms (IBS-C), or functional dyspepsia (FD). One must also take into account the frequency of the symptoms and the degree of dysfunction the patient has (ie, mild annoyance to severe school-absenteeism).

It should be noted that reassurance is a powerful tool. Explaining that while the pain is real, the disorder is not life threatening, and does not progress to other diseases, such as inflammatory bowel disease (IBD) or cancer, is important to emphasize.

One typically needs to address dietary manipulation, largely based on the fact that 60% to 70% of IBS patients believe that certain foods exacerbate their symptoms. Overall, there is insufficient evidence to suggest that exclusion diets are efficacious in FGIDs. Thus, in general, I do not recommend restrictive diets particularly given that in growing children, such diets can lead to significant caloric deprivation and malnutrition. However, an exception to this rule would include a limited trial of 1- to 2-weeks off products containing lactose to distinguish IBS-D from lactose intolerance. If this successfully alleviates all symptoms (in which case the patient does not truly have IBS), patients can then reintroduce lactose-free milk products and/or use lactase supplementation to ensure adequate dietary fat, vitamin D, and calcium. A dietary history should also assess for excessive fructose or sorbitol ingestion and if present, short elimination trials may be helpful. Recent interest in a diet that removes all fermentable foods, called a FODMAP (fermentable oligo-, di-, and monosaccharides and polyols) diet has been shown in a limited number of adults to decrease bloating, pain, nausea, diarrhea, and constipation. Such a diet, however, is very restrictive and should only be considered under the supervision of a dietician. Similarly, the efficacy of a gluten-free diet for presumptive gluten intolerance may be secondary to the elimination of fermentable grains, and a short trial could be considered in patients after the exclusion of celiac disease (CD). I do not recommend fiber supplementation since it has been shown to exacerbate complaints of gas and bloating, even though it may help to improve stool frequency or consistency in patients with IBS-C.

In young children who have relatively mild symptoms, I consider a trial of probiotics as their use appears to be, generally, free of significant side effects. There is some evidence that the intestinal microflora may be altered in patients with IBS, although whether this is causative or an epiphenomenon is unclear. Studies to date have been relatively small but, overall, do seem to help with complaints of abdominal pain and flatulence. I also use probiotics in older children whose parents are reluctant to try medication.

In patients who have episodic pain, typically 2 times per week or less, or those who have predictable triggers, such as a sporting event, I typically use anticholinergic agents. In the United States only 2 such agents are available: hyoscyamine and dicyclomine. A sublingual form of hyoscyamine exists that can typically provide rapid relief within 10 minutes and is my preferred form of medicine for this group of patients. I often make a point to emphasize the rapid onset so as to improve the overall therapeutic effect, and in older children allow a second dose within 15 minutes of the first dose, if needed. Of note, peppermint oil has been shown to act as an antispasmotic as well, and I particularly use this in families who are wary of using medication.

Patients with FD and reflux symptoms often benefit from acid-blockade therapy with a proton pump inhibitor (PPI). PPI therapy may also be helpful in the younger child with RAP who poorly localizes his or her acid-related pain. Cyproheptadine anecdotally also seems helpful for FD patients, particularly those with associated nausea.

For patients with IBS-D, FD, or RAP with more frequent or severe symptoms, I generally prefer the use of tricyclic antidepressants (TCAs). This is largely based on the presumed underlying pathophysiology. I explain that the disease is secondary to dysfunction of the intestinal nerves. These nerves dictate the motility of the intestines, in which rapid transit may contribute to diarrhea. The enteric nerves also alert us to distending pressures; I provide a hypothetical illustration to clarify: If I take a balloon and put it up your bottom (I tell them I will not do this) and inflate the balloon until you feel pain, an IBS or RAP patient will not allow me to inflate the balloon as much as an unaffected child. Adult studies have shown that TCAs are effective in treating the global symptoms of IBS (RR of IBS persisting = 0.68; 95% confidence interval [CI] 0.56 to 0.83). There are 2 pediatric studies, one showing benefit, while the larger, multicenter, randomized, placebo-controlled trial revealed improvement rates similar to placebo, thereby confirming the importance of reassurance and education in treating these disorders. I prefer to use amitriptyline for the IBS-D population as there are some anticholinergic effects that decrease diarrhea. I start with 10 mg and will dose escalate to as high as 1 mg/kg/dose if needed after a 2-week trial. If efficacious, treatment should be a minimum of 2 to 3 months, but longer therapy is often required. The medicine should be taken at night as sleepiness can be a side effect. TCAs can cause prolonged QT, however this is likely a dose-related phenomenon. Routine electrocardiography monitoring is controversial. It is important to mention to parents that though this is an antidepressant, use at low doses (one pill as opposed to 10 to 15 pills) is common for conditions that affect nerves such as pruritis, eneuresis, and nervous bladder. This will avoid phone calls after the patient reads the pharmacy data, and thus may improve adherence. There is also a warning related to suicidality that should be addressed, although likely not an issue in a nondepressed child taking low doses.

Loperamide has been studied in IBS-D; however, it seems to only be effective in decreasing frequency of stooling as opposed to the more global symptoms of pain and bloating. I will rarely use this in patients who claim that stooling urgency is the main problem, as opposed to pain. I also use it on an as needed basis prior to events (ie, school trips and sporting events) where access to the bathroom is likely to be problematic.

The use of nonabsorbable antibiotics for IBS-D has been investigated based on the concept that symptoms are due to either small bowel bacterial overgrowth or the fermentation of nondigested sugars. Adult studies have proven that 10 days of rifaxamin can result in an improvement in a modest percentage of patients. The safety profile makes it a tempting choice for an empiric trial in patients; however, as this is not approved by the Food and Drug Administration (FDA) for use in children and as a costly therapy, it can be difficult to prescribe in children due to the expense. The longevity of the effect and the potential for drug resistance if used chronically over time also are unclear.

The use of laxatives in adolescence with IBS-C has been studied, and while there was no improvement in abdominal pain, stool frequency was increased. I will often use polyethylenegylcol 3350 in IBS-C patients, but it is common that they need other interventions to help with the more global complaints of pain. In those cases, I generally use either a TCA, preferably imipramine or desipramine, which have fewer anticholinergic effects than amitriptyline and are, thus, less constipating, or a selective serotonin reuptake inhibitor (SSRI), which more often has diarrhea as a potential side effect. In adult studies, SSRIs have been shown to improve global IBS symptoms (RR of IBS symptoms persisting = 0.62; 95% CI 0.45 to 0.87).

Lubiprostone is a selective C-2 chloride channel activator. The increase in luminal volume is thought to stimulate colonic motility and improve stool frequency. Studies with IBS-C patients have shown improvement in global symptoms, but there are limited pediatric data.

Cognitive behavioral therapy (CBT) has been proven effective in both adults and children with FGIDs and may be combined with relaxation techniques, parent training, and psychoeducation. For many, CBT is a valuable first-line monotherapy, and it should be emphasized that the techniques one learns through CBT can be used lifelong. Unfortunately, access to psychologists may be limited and costly. I insist on its use in patients who have comorbidities, such as depression or anxiety, although I may combine this with pharmacotherapy to get more rapid symptom relief. SSRIs have greater anxiolytic properties than TCAs, and thus may be preferred in the anxious patient. Although I discourage school absenteeism, I insist on CBT in patients who require limited homeschooling due to severe symptoms.

Finally, it is worth re-emphasizing the placebo rate for FGIDs. This can be as high as 70% and should be used to one's advantage. The physician must reassure the patient that we know the diagnosis, and together we can improve symptoms and quality of life. Parents should be told that distraction from pain is helpful, whereas excessive focusing on the pain is counterproductive. Initially, frequent follow-up is needed to assess symptom relief and medication-related side effects.

Bibliography

American College of Gastroenterology Task Force on Irritable Bowel Syndrome, Brandt LJ, Chey WD, et al. An evidence-based systematic review on the management of irritable bowel syndrome. *Am J Gastroenterol.* 2009;104(suppl 1):S1-S35.

American Academy of Pediatrics Subcommittee on Chronic Abdominal Pain, North American Society for Pediatric Gastroenterology, Hepatology, and Nutrition. Chronic abdominal pain in children. *Pediatrics.* 2005;115:e370-381.

Teitelbaum JE, Arora R. Long-term efficacy of low-dose tricyclic antidepressants for children with functional gastrointestinal disorders. *J Pediatr Gastroenterol Nutr.* 2011;53(3):260-264.

Youssef NN, Rosh JR, Loughran M, et al. Treatment of functional abdominal pain in childhood with cognitive behavioral strategies. *J Pediatr Gastroenterol Nutr.* 2004;39(2):192-196.

37
QUESTION

ACUTE DIARRHEA IS USUALLY INFECTIOUS, BUT WHAT CAUSES RECURRENT OR PERSISTENT DIARRHEA AND HOW SHOULD I EVALUATE SUCH A CONDITION?

Harland Winter, MD

When parents call for the first time to report that their child is having diarrhea, there are some key questions we should ask. Children with diarrhea who have any of the symptoms listed in Table 37-1 should be evaluated by their health care provider.

Diarrhea beginning in the first month of life could be rotavirus, but you should consider dietary protein intolerance or a group of congenital diarrheal disorders that are caused by defects of digestion, absorption, and the transport of nutrients and electrolytes; enterocyte or neuroendocrine defects; or immune deficiencies. In most infants, diarrhea that begins shortly after birth and persists should be evaluated by a pediatric gastroenterologist.[1]

One of the most common causes of persistent or recurrent diarrhea in children is, surprisingly, constipation with encopresis.[2] These children do not appear to be ill, are thriving and growing normally, but may have an increased body mass index and lead a sedentary life. Soiling may be a clue to the diagnosis, but many families just report that their toddler or preschool-aged child is having diarrhea. A careful physical examination with palpation of the left lower quadrant and suprapubic areas to detect palpable stool should reassure you that you are on the right track. However, the best diagnostic test is to place your hand in a glove and carefully do a rectal examination. If done slowly with explanation of what is going to happen, most children can cooperate long enough to get the necessary information. One need only determine if there is stool filling the rectal vault and if the stool is guaiac negative. Feeling a posterior rectal shelf is consistent with chronic constipation. In girls, noting the location of the anus is important as anterior displacement of the anus is more common than in boys. If the anus is closer to the posterior margin of the vagina than it is to the tip of the sacrum, then the rectum may be empty and the stool is more proximal in the colon. A posterior shelf can often be appreciated on examination. For the child who cannot cooperate, the examination should not be performed. Although an abdominal radiograph is not recommended as a diagnostic test for constipation, there are situations when a plain abdominal radiograph is helpful. This is particularly true for

---

Table 37-1
Symptoms in a Child With Diarrhea That Should Prompt an Evaluation By a Health Care Provider

- Fever higher than 102°F
- Diarrhea lasting more than 24 hours
- Dehydration
- Grossly bloody stools (eg, bright-red or maroon blood)
- Melena

---

children with autism who may find it difficult to cooperate with a physical examination; in this group, constipation is a common cause of persistent diarrhea.

Other common conditions that should be considered in the child who is thriving and has a guaiac-negative stool are giardiasis, lactose intolerance (often begins after 7 years of age), drinking a lot of fruit juice, or chewing sugarless gum. Children with persistent diarrhea who have extremely foul-smelling flatus may have giardia, in contrast to children with lactose intolerance who often just have excessive gas. Ordering a lactose breath test is the simplest way to make a diagnosis of lactose intolerance, but remember that children with bacterial overgrowth or an enteropathy secondary to food allergy, a viral infection, or celiac disease (CD) may also be lactose intolerant. A child who is lactose intolerant and has weight loss or growth delay should be evaluated for secondary causes of lactose malabsorption. I usually instruct the family on how to implement a strict lactose-free diet (including milk and casein in cooked foods) for 2 weeks. If the diarrhea resolves with only dietary intervention, a secondary cause is less likely. At this time, I often let the child start to use lactase enzyme supplements when eating foods that contain lactose. Monitoring for abdominal pain, weight loss, and growth delay over time may differentiate other causes of recurrent diarrhea such as irritable bowel syndrome (IBS), which does not affect growth, and development from inflammatory bowel disease (IBD) that often does. Children who have recurrent diarrhea after drinking sucrose-containing foods or beverages should be evaluated for sucrase-isomaltase deficiency by ordering a sucrose breath test or by measuring sucrase-enzyme activity in a duodenal biopsy. If the family has noted that the child gets diarrhea after eating uncooked mushrooms, you may have a patient with a rare trehalase deficiency enabling you to stump all your colleagues at a case conference.

CD is recognized more frequently.[3,4] We used to think of CD presenting in a 1 to 2 year old with chronic diarrhea, irritability, and failure to thrive, but the presentation is changing and this clinical phenotype is not commonly seen. Certainly any child with recurrent or persistent diarrhea should be screened for CD with a serum-IgA (Immunoglobulin A) and IgA-tissue transglutaminase (IgA-tTG). For children younger than 2 years, I usually order an anti-endomysial antibody (anti-EMA) or deamidated gliadin antibodies if these are available. Since about 10% of the population is IgA deficient, they may have a falsely negative IgA-tTG and other diagnostic testing may be needed. An IgG-tTG is available, but if one has a high-suspicion for CD, a duodenal biopsy may be the only way to establish or rule out the diagnosis. Genetic markers—DQ2 and DQ8—are found in about 30% of the general population, but over 98% of patients with CD will have these human leukocyte antigen (HLA) markers. Practically, this means that if a child does not have DQ2 or DQ8, the probability that he or she has CD is extremely small and in most patients a biopsy is not needed; however, if these markers are found and you suspect CD, additional diagnostic studies are warranted.

In addition to carbohydrate malabsorption, persistent diarrhea may also be caused by fat malabsorption. Steatorrhea often results in bulky stools that many families interpret as diarrhea. Sometimes an "oil slick" can be seen on the water in the toilet and the stools may be difficult to flush because they float. This is usually associated with pancreatic insufficiency, most commonly caused in children by cystic fibrosis. However, children who have milder pancreatic insufficiency and neutropenia may have Shwachman's syndrome. Spot stools are not terribly helpful in supporting a diagnosis of steatorrhea, so I rely more on a 72-hour fecal fat with dietary history to calculate the coefficient of absorption.

There are many other causes of recurrent or persistent diarrhea, including antibiotic induced, postinfectious, and diarrhea that is a symptom of an associated chronic illness. Testing the stool for enteric bacterial pathogens and ova/parasites is often an initial part of the evaluation. If blood or white blood cells are found in the stool, colitis should be suspected. There are a few tests one can use to test for polymorphonuclear leucocytes in the stool. In the days of bedside testing, a stool was sent for staining with methylene blue, but now fecal lactoferrin or fecal calprotectin is available. They may be more reliable and can be quantified, but add significant expense to the evaluation. The diagnosis of patients with diarrhea-predominant IBS is made after excluding many other causes of diarrhea, most importantly IBD—Crohn's disease or ulcerative colitis. Children with persistent diarrhea should be evaluated for IBD if they have growth delay, blood or white cells in the stool, weight loss, fevers, recurrent abdominal pain, or delayed puberty. Although about 20% of individuals with IBD will have normal inflammatory markers in the blood, such as c-reactive protein and erythrocyte sedimentation rate, these lab tests along with a complete blood cell count and albumin are often helpful in deciding to refer the patient to a pediatric gastroenterologist.

There are many causes of persistent or recurrent diarrhea and the evaluation may seem complicated. However, there are a few simple observations and tests that will help you begin the work-up. If there is a family history of a chronic illness, be suspicious. Take a dietary history, assess growth and sexual maturation, and perform a physical examination, including a rectal examination. Use this information to decide about sending a stool for ova/parasites, guaiac, and lactoferrin/calprotectin; ordering a lactose breath test or additional lab studies such as celiac serology; or referring the child to a pediatric gastroenterologist.

References

1. Berni Canani R, Terrin G, Cardillo G, Tomaiuolo R, Castaldo G. Congenital diarrheal disorders: improved understanding of gene defects is leading to advances in intestinal physiology and clinical management. *J Pediatr Gastroenterol Nutr.* 2010;50(4):360-366.
2. Constipation Guideline Committee of the North American Society for Pediatric Gastroenterology, Hepatology and Nutrition. Evaluation and treatment of constipation in infants and children: recommendations of the North American Society for Pediatric Gastroenterology, Hepatology and Nutrition. *J Pediatr Gastroenterol Nutr.* 2006;43(3):e1-e13.
3. Rashtak S, Murray JA. Review article: coeliac disease, new approaches to therapy. *Aliment Pharmacol Ther.* 2012;35(7):768-781.
4. Husby S, Koletzko S, Korponay-Szabo IR, et al.; ESPGHAN Working Group on Coeliac Disease Diagnosis; ESPGHAN Gastroenterology Committee; European Society for Pediatric Gastroenterology, Hepatology, and Nutrition. European Society for Pediatric Gastroenterology, Hepatology and Nutrition guidelines for the diagnosis of coeliac disease. *J Pediatr Gastroenterol Nutr.* 2012;54(1):136-160.

38
QUESTION

IS THERE A ROLE FOR PROBIOTICS IN CHILDREN WITH RECURRENT GASTROINTESTINAL SYMPTOMS SUCH AS DIARRHEA OR ABDOMINAL PAIN?

Stefano Guandalini, MD and Catherine D. Newland, MD

When approaching a child with recurrent gastrointestinal (GI) symptoms, such as diarrhea or abdominal pain, the first question you need to ask yourself is, "Are these symptoms caused by a functional or organic process?" Remember, functional means no physiologic, biochemical, or anatomical causes. While in the majority of cases these issues are part of the very common functional GI disorders, in some cases they may be an expression of an underlying disease that needs to be addressed. Thus, you may first want to consider in your differential diagnosis the causes listed in Table 38-1. An intelligent and expedited use of a few tests, especially when in the presence of one or more red flags (see Table 38-1), will typically suffice to rule out these conditions and conclude for a functional disorder. With symptoms likely caused by a functional process, this is when your attention should turn to the possible use of probiotics.

Probiotics are defined as healthy bacteria and living organisms, usually bacteria or yeast, that when ingested in adequate amounts are beneficial to the patient. The use of probiotics has become an increasingly popular trend in the United States during recent years, and they are now widely available in health food stores, pharmacies, and grocery stores in the form of yogurts, dairy products, health bars, and supplements. The global probiotic market has generated billions of dollars per year and there are hundreds of products available for purchase. Parents are often enthusiastic about using natural or organic alternatives and may ask your opinion about which probiotics are safe to use, even in healthy children. These factors, along with the growing list of touted health benefits—from improving diarrhea to treating allergies—can make prescribing probiotics a daunting task.

In the past 15 to 20 years, there has been a rush for scientists and clinicians to investigate how probiotics work, which organisms are truly beneficial, and for what conditions. Despite the focus, the mechanism of action for probiotics is not completely clear, and it is likely that different strains will have different mechanisms. Overall, they are thought to keep pathogenic organisms in check, improve the intestinal-barrier function, and play a role in immune function.

We always emphasize with our patients that not all probiotics are created equal. Many readily-available preparations have not been studied and have no proven efficacy. However, the formulations that have been found to be beneficial can indeed have an impact on a patient's health. Parents often

Table 38-1

Common Organic Causes of Recurrent Diarrhea and/or Abdominal Pain in Children

Condition	Red Flags	Useful Screening Diagnostic Tools
Intestinal infections	History of recent travels Use of well water Recent onset Other household members affected Associated vomiting, fever, and hematochezia	Stool tests for O&P Stool culture (include *Clostridium difficile*) Search for rotavirus, norovirus, Adenovirus 20, 21
IBD	Hematochezia Systemic signs/symptoms • Fatigue • Weight loss • Joint pain • Night sweats • Skin rashes Abdominal exam • Localized tenderness • Mass	CBC with differential CRP, ESR Fecal calprotectin
CD	Family history of celiac disease or other autoimmune conditions Systemic signs/symptoms • Fatigue • Weight loss or failure to thrive • Joint pain Abdominal exam • Distention	tTG DGP Total serum-IgA
Eosinophilic gastroenteropathy	Associated food allergies Associated vomiting and hematochezia Anemia Peripheral eosinophilia Weight loss	CBC with differential Serum albumin Fecal hemoccult Fecal alpha-1-anti-trypsin Fecal calprotectin
Helicobactor pylori gastritis	Associated dyspeptic symptoms Vomiting Abdominal exam • Tenderness in epigastric area	Fecal *H pylori* antigen test

IBD: irritable bowel disease; CD: celiac disease; O&P: ova and parasite CBC: complete blood cell count; CRP: C-reactive protein; ESR: erythrocyte sedimentation rate; tTG: tissue transglutaminase antibodies; DGP: deamidated gliadin peptides.

ask if eating yogurt is an adequate substitute for taking a probiotic formulation. Unfortunately, the bacterial strains that are used in most of the unpasteurized yogurts available do not have the same favorable effects as some of the commercially-available products: their concentrations are manifold lower and may not survive the acidic environment of the stomach as readily.

The use of probiotics in the treatment of acute infectious diarrhea has been studied extensively. A meta-analysis by Allen et al[1] showed that probiotics reduce the duration of diarrhea by about 24 hours, reduce the risk of diarrhea lasting more than 4 days, and decrease the number of stools by the second day of illness. This study showed there were no adverse events when using probiotics. *Lactobacillus GG* and *Saccharomyces boulardii* have been the most widely studied strains and are thought to be the most efficacious in acute diarrheal illness. In our practice, we typically recommend the use of one of these strains at the onset of a diarrheal illness in conjunction with oral rehydration therapy. The minimal effective dose seems to be 10 billion colony-forming units and should ideally be given within the first 48 hours of illness. Probiotics, particularly *Lactobacillus GG*, may also have the ability to decrease shedding of rotavirus, which would reduce the risk of spreading the illness.

Probiotics may also play an important role in preventing the onset of antibiotic-associated diarrhea. Systematic reviews indicate that taking a probiotic while on antibiotic treatment may decrease the incidence of diarrhea. If your patient is about to begin a course of antibiotics (especially one known to cause diarrhea), it may be worthwhile prescribing a probiotic; the same applies to patients who have previously experienced antibiotic-associated diarrhea. Guandalini et al[2] summarized the evidence of using probiotics in cases of diarrhea.

If your assessment is that the child for whom you are providing care has recurrent diarrhea as a part of irritable syndrome (ie, if you conclude that he or she has functional recurrent abdominal pain associated with functional diarrhea), then probiotics may be beneficial. Recurrent abdominal pain is indeed a disturbing ailment that leaves clinicians looking for an ideal treatment, particularly given the lack of safe and effective drugs. A meta-analysis of 16 randomized-controlled trials[3] showed *Bifidobacterium infantis* may be effective in reducing symptoms of irritable bowel syndrome (IBS), but many of the other study results were limited by their methodology. We recently published results of a multicenter study that looked at the efficacy of the probiotic VSL#3 in alleviating IBS-related symptoms (abdominal pain, bloating, and stool dysfunction) in children and teenaged patients. We found this probiotic safe and significantly more effective than the placebo in treating IBS symptoms and improving quality of life.[4] Therefore, we feel this safe preparation could be a useful tool when used in combination with proper medical care, including reassurance and a caring follow-up.

Probiotics are available as dietary supplements and come in a variety of forms, including capsules, tablets, sachets, and powders. No prescription is required, but it is important to emphasize with patients the formulation that has been shown to be helpful for their specific condition. Most are recommended to be taken once daily for maximum benefit and there are no known safety concerns with prolonged use. The satchel or powder forms can be easily opened and mixed with cold food, like applesauce or ice cream, for younger patients. Capsules are easily opened for mixing.

Probiotics are generally considered to be safe. If you think about the normal bowel, there are more than 100 trillion micro-organisms and most probiotics contain the same type of organisms that are found in a healthy GI tract. Most have no side effects that are different from taking a placebo and can be safely taken with other medications and vitamins. Please note that some probiotics may contain dairy, gluten, and other additives of which patients with allergies or celiac disease (CD) need to be aware. Caution should be taken in administering probiotics in critically ill and immunocompromised patients. Concern has been specifically raised about using *Saccharomyces boulardii* in the presence of a central venous catheter.

Depending on the type of probiotic, it may be regulated by the Food and Drug Administration (FDA) as a dietary supplement, a food, or a drug. Keep in mind that probiotics that are not

Table 38-2
Probiotics Recommended for Diarrhea and/or Abdominal Pain in Children

Brand Name	Strain	Uses	Comments	Approximate Pricing
Florastor	*Saccharomyces boulardii* (yeast)	Antibiotic-associated diarrhea	No refrigeration needed Gluten free Contraindicated if central line or yeast allergy	20 packets for $20.99
VSL#3	*Bifidobacterium* (breve, longum, infantis) *Lactobacillus* (acidophilus, plantarum, Paracasei, bulgaricus) *Streptococcus* (thermophilus)	IBS UC Ileal "pouchitis"	Requires refrigeration (lasts 1 week without refrigeration) Mix with cold water or cold food	30 sachets for $86.00
Culturelle	*Lactobacillus rhamnosus GG*	Acute infectious diarrhea Antibiotic-associated diarrhea	Store at room temperature or refrigerate Take with or without food	30 packets for $26.99
Align	*Bifidobacterium infantis* 35624	IBS	Store at room temperature Take with water, with or without food	28 capsules for $29.99

IBS: irritable bowel syndrome; UC: ulcerative colitis.

approved by the FDA as a drug are oftentimes not covered by insurance. The cost of using a probiotic on a daily basis may, therefore, be a barrier to its use. We often suggest that our patients buy the product online where it can often be found at a lower price. Table 38-2 lists probiotics and their indications. Not all patients will benefit from probiotics, and if they have seen no change in their symptoms after several weeks of treatment, there is no reason to continue use.

Given the positive evidence and minimal risk, we feel it is appropriate to consider using probiotics as adjuvant therapy in acute infectious diarrhea, antibiotic-associated diarrhea, and IBS. Continued research is necessary to further define other health conditions that may benefit from probiotics, the most efficacious strains, optimal dosage, and length of treatment.

References

1. Allen SJ, Martinez EG, Gregorio GV, Dans LF. Probiotics for treating acute infectious diarrhoea. *Cochrane Database Syst Rev.* 2010;(11):CD003048.
2. Guandalini S, Magazzu A, Chiaro A, et al. VSL#3 improves symptoms in children with irritable bowel syndrome: a multicenter, randomized, placebo-controlled, double-blind, crossover study. *J Pediatr Gastroenterol Nutr.* 2010;51(1):24-30.
3. Guandalini S. Probiotics for prevention and treatment of diarrhea. *J Clin Gastroenterol.* 2011;45(suppl):S149-X153.
4. Brenner DM, Moeller MJ, Chey WD, Shoenfeld PS. The utility of probiotics in the treatment of irritable bowel syndrome: a systematic review. *Am J Gastroenterol.* 2009;104(4):1033-1049.

SECTION VIII

INFLAMMATORY
BOWEL DISEASE

What Is the Current Understanding of the Etiology of Inflammatory Bowel Disease?

Lindsey Albenberg, DO and Robert N. Baldassano, MD

Crohn's disease and ulcerative colitis (UC) are inflammatory bowel diseases (IBD) that result in chronic, relapsing inflammation of the gastrointestinal (GI) tract. The pathogenesis of these disorders is complex and a specific etiology has not been elucidated. The available evidence suggests that IBD involves an abnormal immune response, likely to environmental factors, in a genetically susceptible host.[1] In fact, there has been an increase in disease prevalence during the past 4 decades that is hypothesized to be, at least in part, secondary to these environmental factors. Many of the implicated nongenetic factors, such as diet and antibiotic use, have a clear effect on the intestinal micro-organism flora or the gut microbiota. This is understandable as host-microbe interactions are believed to play an important role in the pathogenesis of these diseases.

It is now generally accepted that IBD results from an abnormal inflammatory response to intestinal bacteria. Murine models of colitis, for example, require intestinal bacteria in order to demonstrate inflammation.[2] Germ-free mice with genetic defects, which typically lead to colitis, do not, in fact, develop colitis.[2] Clinically, there is also significant evidence to support the relationship between the gut microbiota and IBD. For example the inflammation in both Crohn's disease and UC occurs predominately in the terminal ileum and colon, where the greatest concentrations of bacteria are found.[2] In addition, antibiotics, such as metronidazole and ciprofloxacin, can be a modestly effective treatment for Crohn's disease. It is important to recognize that there are trillions of organisms that live in the human gut and more than 1000 species; however, no specific pathogen has been implicated in the development of IBD. Multiple studies have evaluated the role of specific bacteria in the development of IBD, such as *Myobacterium avium* subspecies *paratuberculosis* (MAP); however, these studies have been inconclusive.[3] Rather, in IBD, it is thought that the normal bacteria in the gut activate the immune response and provide constant immune system stimulation.

In terms of the intestinal immune system, a delicate balance exists. It is important for the host immune system to tolerate commensal intestinal micro-organisms and protect against potential pathogens. IBD develops when alterations in this balance occur. The pathogenesis of IBD is believed to involve both the innate and the adaptive immune systems.[1] Recall that the innate immune system is nonspecific and represents our first line of defense against pathogens. The innate immune system comprises neutrophils, macrophages, dendritic cells, and natural-killer T-cells. In IBD, there is an infiltration of innate immune system cells into the lamina propria of the intestine. The innate immune system then primes the adaptive immune system.[1] The adaptive immune system, conversely, is antigen-specific, and the response is not mobilized immediately. Lymphocytes, such as B-cells and T-cells, are responsible for this portion of the immune response. In IBD, there is an exaggerated T-cell response. More specifically, there is activation of certain CD 4+ T-helper cells, including T-helper 1 cells (Th1), T-helper 2 cells (Th2), and T-helper 17 cells (Th17). Over activity of these T-helper cells results in poorly regulated secretion of pro-inflammatory cytokines. Examples of these cytokines include the tumor necrosis factor alpha (TNF-α), interleukin-1β, interferon γ, and cytokines of the interleukin 23-Th 17 pathway. In IBD, it is thought that the immune system's abnormal response to enteric flora causes an imbalance in the cytokine production profile at different points throughout the disease process.[4,5] These cytokines have been an important target for therapies. Most notable are the anti-TNF-α medications, such as infliximab.

Genetic studies have also demonstrated the importance of the relationship between the host and commensal bacteria. There is clearly a genetic role in both Crohn's disease and UC. However, the influence of genetics appears to be greater in Crohn's disease than in UC, with cumulative monozygotic twin concordance rates of 36% and 16%, respectively.[6] Recent genome-wide association studies utilizing high-density single-nucleotide polymorphism array technology has identified greater than 100 loci associated with Crohn's disease and UC, both of which involve the innate and the adaptive immune system.[7]

An example of this relationship between genetics and the abnormal immune system response to commensal bacteria in IBD is seen in the association between mutations of the nucleotide-binding oligomerization domain-containing protein 2 (NOD-2) gene and Crohn's disease. The NOD-2 gene encodes a protein that senses peptidoglycan, a component of the bacterial-cell wall.[1] There are many theories regarding how mutations in the NOD-2 gene contribute to the inflammation of Crohn's disease, but it is thought to involve abnormalities in the innate immune system. No theory has been universally accepted and this remains an active area of research. Interestingly, studies of patients with Crohn's disease suggest a relationship between polymorphisms in the NOD-2 gene and Crohn's disease phenotype. Specifically, patients who have fibrostenotic disease of the terminal ileum requiring intestinal resection may have a higher incidence of NOD-2 mutations.[1]

There are many other genes that have been linked to the pathogenesis of Crohn's disease and UC; these diseases are believed to be polygenic. Still, it is believed that known genetic associations account for only 20% of the genetic variance in IBD.[1] These are complex disorders that involve nongenetic factors. It is also assumed that there are remaining genetic factors that have not yet been identified. The field is advancing quickly in this area and our knowledge of the pathogenesis of IBD will without a doubt continue to grow in the coming years.

References

1. Abraham C, Cho JH. Inflammatory bowel disease. *N Engl J Med*. 2009;361(21):2066-2078.
2. Sartor RB. Microbial influences in inflammatory bowel diseases. *Gastroenterology*. 2008;134(2):577-594.
3. Flanagan P, Campbell BJ, Rhodes JM. Bacteria in the pathogenesis of inflammatory bowel disease. *Biochem Soc Trans*. 2011;39(4):1067-1072.
4. Alex P, Zachos N, Nguyen T, et al. Distinct cytokine patterns identified from multiplex profiles of murine DSS and TNBS-induced colitis. *Inflamm Bowel Dis*. 2009;15(3):341-352.
5. Blumberg RS. Inflammation in the intestinal tract: pathogenesis and treatment. *Dig Dis*. 2009;27(4):455-464.
6. Russell RK, Satsangi J. IBD: a family affair. *Best Pract Res Clin Gastroenterol*. 2004;18(3):525-539.
7. Shikhare G, Kugathasan S. Inflammatory bowel disease in children: current trends. *J Gastroenterol*. 2010;45(7): 673-682.

HOW ARE THE DIFFERENT TYPES OF INFLAMMATORY BOWEL DISEASE DIAGNOSED AND CLASSIFIED?

Jeremy P. Middleton, MD and Subra Kugathasan, MD

The simplest way to think about inflammatory bowel disease (IBD) in children is to classify patients as having either Crohn's disease or ulcerative colitis (UC). Fitting children into one of these categories is important since the natural history and potential treatment strategies are different for each. Furthermore, children must have a definitive diagnosis of Crohn's disease or UC to enter into research studies, including clinical trials. Once given a diagnosis of Crohn's disease or UC, we can further classify these children based on their phenotype.

UC classification depends on disease location. Proctitis is limited to the rectum; left-sided colitis extends just past the splenic flexure; subtotal colitis extends past the hepatic flexure; and pancolitis involves the entire large bowel from the cecum to the rectum. Crohn's disease is subclassified based on disease behavior and is described as either inflammatory, stricturing, or penetrating. Patients with each of these subclasses of Crohn's disease can have perianal disease, making it a modifier of each classification, rather than a class in and of itself. Some patients with disease isolated to the colon can have characteristics of both Crohn's disease and UC. Comprising almost 10% to 20% of newly diagnosed children, we refer to this group as having colonic IBD, type unclassified (IBDU). Some believe that IBDU is a separate condition entirely, while others feel that, with time, a child's clinical course will point more toward a diagnosis of Crohn's disease or UC. Although there is still debate about the definition, diagnosis, and treatment of IBDU, we always reassure parents and patients that because the treatment strategies are so similar, the title of the diagnosis is not as important. Fortunately, we can diagnose the majority of patients as having either Crohn's disease or UC. Because this distinction is so important, pediatric gastroenterologists use not only signs, symptoms, and laboratory findings at initial evaluation but a variety of diagnostic tools that can delineate these 2 classifications.

Before we can classify a child as having Crohn's disease or UC, we must first determine which children have IBD. Although children with IBD present with a variety of different clinical manifestations, the most common presentation is abdominal pain and bloody diarrhea. Since infectious colitis causes these same symptoms, it is imperative to rule out infection. A child who complains of such red-flag symptoms as isolated right lower quadrant pain, nocturnal stooling, nighttime abdominal pain, unexplained fever, or weight loss warrants further laboratory evaluation. Although 20% of children with IBD have normal lab work, the presence of hypoal-buminemia, anemia, thrombocytosis, and/or elevated inflammatory markers is common in IBD, making a comprehensive metabolic panel, CBC with differential, erythrocyte sedimentation rate (ESR), and c-reactive protein (CRP) good screening-tests (Table 40-1). Once we are convinced that a child is likely to have IBD, we then focus on determining which type of IBD is present.

We can never give a child a diagnosis of Crohn's disease or UC based only on their signs, symptoms, or laboratory findings alone. There are certain features, though, that can sway us more toward a diagnosis of Crohn's disease. Children with Crohn's disease more frequently present with oral aphthous ulcers, upper gastrointestinal (GI) complaints, persistent unexplained fever, poor growth, delayed puberty, or perianal disease. There are also certain extra-intestinal manifestations seen more often in one type of IBD than another. Children with Crohn's disease are more likely to have joint disease and erythema nodosum, while in UC, primary sclerosing cholangitis and pyoderma gangrenosum is more common. Even though a higher percentage of children with Crohn's disease have hypoalbuminemia and an elevated ESR, these findings are not specific to Crohn's disease (see Table 40-1). Unfortunately none of these symptoms, physical-exam findings, extra-intestinal manifestations, or laboratory results are exclusive to one type of IBD versus another, so further evaluation is always necessary to make a specific diagnosis.

Although children with IBD have a chronic inflammatory condition, many acute conditions, like infection, can mimic the signs and symptoms of IBD. Our first job is to determine whether there is a chronic component of the inflammation making endoscopy with biopsy the gold stan-dard of IBD diagnostic testing. Histology is the best way to determine if inflammation or ulcer-ation seen endoscopically is due to a chronic process rather than an acute illness. Endoscopy not only obtains pathologic specimens for histologic review, but evaluating the patterns of inflam-mation can help differentiate Crohn's disease from UC. Children with UC have inflammation limited to the colon, while in Crohn's disease the inflammation can be anywhere in the GI tract. Endoscopically, the inflammation in UC is continuous and superficial starting in the rectum and spreading proximally (Figure 40-1A). Crohn's disease inflammation appears as discrete aphthous or deep-linear ulcers with cobblestoning of the mucosa (Figure 40-1B). A child with Crohn's disease will have patchy inflammation with areas of healthy mucosa in between areas of disease. Colonoscopy with ileal intubation is paramount in diagnosing IBD since small-bowel involvement is highly suggestive of Crohn's disease (see Table 40-1). Initial evaluation of IBD also includes assessment of the upper GI tract with esophagogastroduodenoscopy (EGD). We can give parents a confident diagnosis of Crohn's disease if there are aphthous ulcers in the stomach or duodenum with granulomas seen on biopsy (the pathognomonic histologic finding of Crohn's disease).

Sometimes the endoscopy can be deceiving. Nonspecific gastric or duodenal inflammation can be seen in both Crohn's disease and UC. Even though Crohn's disease is typically the culprit when there is small bowel disease, a small percentage of patients with UC have mild terminal ileum inflammation termed *backwash ileitis*. If after endoscopy and review of the histology we are still unable to differentiate Crohn's disease from UC, we have several tools that can help make a diagnosis.

Radiographic evaluation in children with IBD is integral in evaluating the location, extent, and severity of disease. If these studies show small bowel disease, narrowing from stricture, fistula, or perianal disease, we can confidently make a diagnosis of Crohn's disease. A variety of radiographic techniques have been employed in evaluating children with IBD, including contrast studies, com-puterized tomography (CT), and magnetic resonance imaging (MRI). An upper GI with small bowel follow through can show areas of small intestine inflammation, narrowing, and/or presence of fistula. Imaging of the bowel with CT not only identifies acute and chronic inflammation of the small bowel and colon, but also characterizes complications of Crohn's disease, such as abscess formation, fistula, and perianal disease. Due to concerns about radiation exposure with repeat imaging performed on patients with IBD, MRI is becoming more appealing than fluoroscopy or

Table 40-1

Differences Between Crohn's Disease and Ulcerative Colitis

	Crohn's Disease	*UC*
Clinical Features and Labs at Presentation (% of patients)		
Abdominal pain	65 to 70	40 to 70
Diarrhea	30 to 55	75 to 95
Bleeding	20 to 40	80
Weight loss	55 to 60	30 to 40
Fatigue	10 to 30	2 to 12
Anorexia	25	6
Arthritis	1 to 7	6
Nausea/vomiting	6	0.5
Perianal disease	6	0
Growth failure/delayed puberty	4	0
Anemia	16 to 77	30
Hypoalbuminemia	35 to 64	15
Elevated ESR	85	23
Elevated CRP	>90	85
Endoscopy		
Extent of inflammation	Anywhere in the GI tract	Limited to colon
Pattern of inflammation	"Patchy" with normal mucosa in between diseased tissue (skip lesions); associated with rectal sparing	Diffuse; generally begins at the rectum and spreads proximally; often with an abrupt transition from diseased to normal appearing tissue
Appearance of inflammation	Discrete aphthous ulcers; linear ulcers causing cobblestoning; deep ulcers	Erythema; loss of vascular pattern; friability; superficial ulcers
Imaging		
Upper GI with small bowel follow through	Identifies ulcers, narrowing, and fistula in the small bowel	Normal small bowel

(continued)

Table 40-1 (continued)

Differences between Crohn's Disease and Ulcerative Colitis

	Crohn's Disease	*UC*
CT	Identifies small bowel wall edema, mesenteric/creeping fat, fluid collections, stricture, fistula, and perianal disease	Thickening of the colon with "lead pipe" appearance
MRI	Identifies small bowel wall edema, mesenteric/creeping fat, fluid collections, stricture, fistula, and perianal disease without radiation	Thickening of the colon with "lead pipe" appearance
Video Capsule Endoscopy	Documents presence and extent of inflammation and ulceration in the small bowel	Limited role in UC
Serology (% of patients)		
ASCA	40 to 80	< 10
pANCA	10 to 27 (typically, colonic CD)	60 to 80

CD: Crohn's disease; ESR: erythrocyte sedimentation rate; CSR: C-reactive protein; GI: gastrointestinal; CT: computerized tomography; MRI: magnetic resonance imaging; ASCA: erevisiae antibody; pANCA: perinuclear anti-nuclear cytoplasmic antibody.

CT due to its lack of harmful ionizing radiation. Although not as readily available and at times requiring sedation, MRI is excellent at evaluating the bowel wall for acute and chronic inflammation, identifying fistula, and assessing perianal disease (Figure 40-1D).

Radiographic studies are great noninvasive methods of evaluating the bowel, but there is no better way to evaluate the small bowel mucosa than with direct visualization using either video capsule endoscopy (VCE) or small bowel enteroscopy. We have been using VCE for the last decade to document the presence of inflammation or ulcers in the small bowel. The device, a large pill-sized capsule with a camera, light source, and radio transmitter, is either swallowed or deployed endoscopically. The camera takes a picture every half second as it travels through the GI tract, enabling visualization of subtle mucosal abnormalities that cross-sectional imaging may miss (Figure 40-1C). Although VCE is a very safe procedure, there is about a 2% risk of pill retention. Preprocedure capsule patency tests minimize, but cannot eliminate, this risk. Small bowel enteroscopy is an endoscopic technique enabling evaluation of a large portion of the small intestines. There is special equipment and additional training necessary to perfect this technique and many centers may not have access to small bowel enteroscopy.

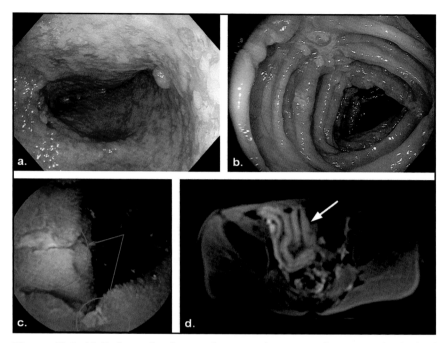

Figure 40-1. (a) Endoscopic picture of severe ulcerative colitis. Note the lack of vascular pattern and diffuse erythema and ulceration. There is a single inflammatory polyp at the 2 o'clock position often seen in ulcerative colitis. (b) Endoscopic picture of a linear ulcer in Crohn's disease. Notice that there is relatively healthy tissue surrounding the ulcer. (c) Capsule endoscopy picture of 2 deep, aphthous ulcers in a patient with Crohn's disease. (d) MRI showing active inflammation with terminal ileum thickening and edema in a patient with Crohn's disease.

Certain serologic markers are seen more frequently in patients with each type of IBD. These markers are poor screening tests, although many practitioners utilize them to help differentiate Crohn's disease from UC. Unfortunately, we have found them less helpful in making this distinction. Although a majority of patients with a positive perinuclear anti-neutrophil cytoplasmic antibody (pANCA) have UC, there is a percentage of patients with colonic Crohn's disease who are also pANCA positive. Anti-*Saccharomyces cerevisiae* antibody (ASCA) is seen in 40% to 80% of patients with Crohn's disease, but many of these ASCA positive patients have isolated small bowel disease where the diagnosis of Crohn's disease is already certain (see Table 40-1). Research suggests that these types of serologic markers may play an important role in predicting the severity of a patient's disease course, but we find them infrequently helpful in differentiating Crohn's disease from UC.

Although the cause of IBD is yet unknown, there are definite genetic and environmental factors involved. The future of IBD diagnosis and classification will likely be evaluating a patient's genome for particular polymorphisms that are associated with Crohn's disease or UC. This is already happening with a commercially available test that uses the presence of nucleotide-binding oligomerization domain-containing protein 2 (NOD2)/caspase recruitment domain gene (CARD15) polymorphisms to help predict disease. NOD2/CARD15 mutations are present in approximately one-quarter of White patients with Crohn's disease and are associated with ileal disease that is likely to progress to a more complicated disease course. We believe, at present, that genetic markers should not be used to diagnose or prognosticate an individual, but rather be reserved for investigational purposes only. We do believe computer algorithms that combine genetics, serology, and microbial markers will be used in the near future to develop prediction models for accurate diagnosis and prognosis in Crohn's disease and UC.

It is important that we give children with IBD a diagnosis of Crohn's disease or UC. Although initial evaluation with a thorough physical examination, screening laboratory results, and stool studies can help determine if a child is likely to have IBD, we rely on endoscopy, radiographic studies, and direct visualization techniques to provide an accurate diagnosis of Crohn's disease or UC. Due to the poor sensitivity of the serologic markers, we feel they are not helpful in screening children for IBD and are not very reliable in differentiating Crohn's disease from UC. Though the future is in genetic screening, we are uncertain of the utility of available testing. IBD is a lifelong, chronic inflammatory condition and we feel that children with symptoms of IBD should be diagnosed only after careful evaluation by a pediatric gastroenterologist.

Bibliography

Mamula P, Markowitz JE, Baldassano RN. *Pediatric Inflammatory Bowel Disease*. NY: Springer; 2007.

North American Society for Pediatric Gastroenterology, Hepatology, and Nutrition, Colitis Foundation of America; Bousvaros A, Antonioli DA, Colletti RB, et al. Differentiating ulcerative colitis from Crohn disease in children and young adults: report of a working group of the North American Society for Pediatric Gastroenterology, Hepatology, and Nutrition and the Crohn's and Colitis Foundation of America. *J Pediatr Gastroenterol Nutr.* 2007;44(5):653-674.

Silverberg MS, Satsangi J, Ahmad T, et al. Toward an integrated clinical, molecular and serological classification of inflammatory bowel disease: Report of a Working Party of the 2005 Montreal World Congress of Gastroenterology. *Can J Gastroenterol.* 2005;19(suppl A):5-36.

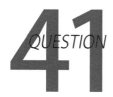

ARE THERE NEW CLASSES OF INFLAMMATORY BOWEL DISEASE THERAPIES OF WHICH I SHOULD BE AWARE?

Bella Zeisler, MD and Jeffrey S. Hyams, MD

Until the 1990s, the treatment of pediatric inflammatory bowel disease (IBD) was largely dependent upon corticosteroids and sulfasalazine. As the efficacy of sulfasalazine was limited, particularly for patients with Crohn's disease, long-term corticosteroid exposure was common resulting in hypertension, psychiatric difficulties, as well as other known corticosteroid side effects. Nutritional support was common either with nasogastric tube feedings or total parental nutrition. It was clear that patient quality of life was often poor.

As treatment strategies for IBD evolved in the 1990s, immunomodulators, including thiopurines (6-mercaptopurine and its pro-drug azathioprine), were increasingly employed for corticosteroid-dependent patients. In the year 2000, data were published showing that the introduction of thiopurines at diagnosis in children with moderate to severe Crohn's disease was associated with better outcomes.[1] More recently, thiopurines have also been shown to be of benefit in the treatment of moderate to severe ulcerative colitis (UC) not responsive to 5-aminosalicylates.[2] It is important to point out that thiopurines may take up to 3 to 4 months to start working, so they have little role in patients with active disease who are corticosteroid refractory. Although thiopurines are most often well tolerated, there are a host of potential side effects (some severe) that need to be kept in mind, and patients on these medications need to be monitored vigilantly. Severe side effects can include pancreatitis, allergic reactions, and leukopenia due to bone marrow suppression. A 4-fold increase over baseline in the incidence of non-Hodgkin's lymphoma has been reported in adults. There also appears to be an increase in nonmelanoma skin cancers. An extremely rare but aggressive and almost universally fatal malignancy called hepatosplenic T-cell lymphoma has been associated with thiopurine use either alone or in combination with anti-tumor necrosis factor alpha (TNF-α) therapy.[3] This rare malignancy is much more common in males than in females, especially during the teenaged and early-adulthood years.

More recently, methotrexate has been increasingly used for patients with moderate to severe Crohn's disease either as a first-line agent instead of thiopurines, or when thiopurines fail or are not well tolerated.[4] Methotrexate is a structural analog of folic acid that acts by inhibiting the metabolism of folic acid. Although the cellular action of methotrexate is well understood, the mechanism by which it improves symptoms of IBD remains unclear. Methotrexate is likely to be more efficacious when given via subcutaneous injection but may also be given orally. Possible adverse effects include ulcerative stomatitis, leukopenia, increased risk for infection, nausea, abdominal pain, fatigue, fever, dizziness, and rarely pulmonary fibrosis and hepatitis. Methotrexate is highly teratogenic and categorized as pregnancy category X by the Food and Drug Administration (FDA). Women must not take the drug during pregnancy, if there is a risk of becoming pregnant, or if they are breastfeeding. Therefore, this drug is generally not felt to be a good option for teenaged females of childbearing age. As methotrexate has had no association with hepatosplenic T-cell lymphoma, its use as the immunodulator of choice in young males has increased. It should be noted that males who plan to father a child should consider stopping the medication several months before attempting fertilization.

Biologic agents that have been used for the treatment of several autoimmune disorders, including psoriasis, ankylosing spondylitits, psoriatic arthritis, and rheumatoid arthritis, are the newest class of drugs indicated for the treatment of moderate to severe IBD. Infliximab was the first biologic agent used for treatment of IBD, having received initial FDA approval in 1998 for adults with Crohn's disease and subsequently for UC. It was approved for pediatric Crohn's disease in 2006 and pediatric UC in 2011. Infliximab is generally indicated for the induction of remission as well as the maintenance of remission for moderate to severe disease, and is often used as a first line in Crohn's disease characterized by extensive small bowel involvement, fistulae, or growth-restricting disease.[5] Infliximab is a chimeric monoclonal antibody (70% human, 30% mouse) against TNF-α, which is a proinflammatory molecule. Although rare, serious and sometimes fatal side effects have been documented with the use of infliximab, including serious blood dyscrasias, and infections including reactivation of hepatitis B or tuberculosis, lymphoma, drug-induced lupus, demylelinating central nervous system disorders, liver injury, and solid-tissue cancers. Hepatosplenic T-cell lymphoma has also been associated with infliximab when used in combination with a thiopurine. Patients receiving infliximab must be screened regularly for the development of these possible complications. During the first years after approval by the FDA, infliximab was often used on an intermittent/sporadic schedule. However, it has been more recently discovered that maintenance therapy with regularly-scheduled infusions decreases the likelihood of developing antibodies to infliximab that are known to reduce the efficacy of the drug. Infliximab is administered intravenously generally every 8 weeks following 3 loading doses.

Subsequent to FDA approval of infliximab, other biologic agents have gained approval in adults for the treatment of IBD. Adalimumab, FDA approved for adult patients in 2007, is a fully humanized anti-TNF alpha monoclonal antibody that has been shown to be efficacious in the treatment of moderate to severely ill children with Crohn's disease, whether they are anti-TNF naive or experienced.[6] Rather than intravenous delivery, adalimumab is injected subcutaneously every other week or in some cases every week, typically by the patient at home. Certolizumab pegol, another biologic agent, was FDA approved in 2008 for the induction and maintenance of remission in adults with moderate to severe IBD who did not show adequate response to other standard therapies, including infliximab or adalimumab. This agent is a PEGylated (ie, attached to polyethylene glycol) antigen binding fragment (Fab) of a humanized TNF inhibitor that is administered subcutaneously every 4 weeks after 3 induction doses are given. The linked polyethylene glycol is felt to increase the plasma half life, reducing the need for frequent dosing and, thus, possibly reducing immunogenicity. In addition, certolizumab does not cross the placenta and has been used throughout pregnancy in adult patients. Natalizumab, another biologic agent, is a humanized monoclonal antibody to alpha 4 integrin, a cell adhesion molecule. By blocking the activity of alpha 4 integrin, natalizumab is thought to inhibit leukocyte migration from the blood vessels to sites of inflammation. It is used in patients with moderate to severe Crohn's disease, refractory to other standard forms of medical therapy. It is given by intravenous infusion every 4 weeks. Natalizumab was FDA approved in 2004 but was subsequently withdrawn from the market by its manufacturer after it was linked with cases of the rare neurological condition progressive multifocal leukoencephalopathy (PML) caused by the John Cunningham virus. It was then reintroduced to the United States market in 2006 under a restricted distribution program. As of January 2010, there have been 31 cases of PML associated with natalizumab therapy.

In addition to the major classes of medications used for the treatment of pediatric IBD discussed previously, there are several additional therapies less frequently employed. Elemental or polymeric formulas delivered orally or via nasogastric tube may be beneficial for induction and maintenance of remission in inflammatory Crohn's disease when used as the exclusive or predominant form of nutrition. While its use has not been widespread in the United States likely due to cultural and patient preference factors, this form of therapy is more commonly used in parts of Europe. In addition, there is evidence to suggest that under certain circumstances, probiotics may be beneficial, such as the use of VSL#3 for the prevention of recurrent pouchitis in patients who have undergone ileal pouch-anal anastomosis surgery. Finally, antibiotics such as metronidazole and ciprofloxacin, which are also felt to have additional anti-inflammatory properties, are sometimes used as adjunctive intermittent therapy, particularly in Crohn's disease with perianal involvement.

At present, there are a handful of classes of medications available for the treatment of pediatric IBD. Choice of treatment will depend on a variety of factors, including severity, distribution/location of disease, whether the patient's disease is classified as Crohn's disease or UC, age, and gender of the patient. Additional patient factors that need to be considered when prescribing treatment for IBD include personal preference of the patient and family, and the patient's ability to maintain adherence to sometimes complicated regimens.

References

1. Markowitz J, Grancher K, Kohn N, Lesser M, Daum F. A multicenter trial of 6-mercaptopurine and prednisone in children with newly diagnosed Crohn's disease. *Gastroenterology.* 2000;119(4):895-902.
2. Hyams JS, Lerer T, Mack D, et al; Pediatric Inflammatory Bowel Disease Collaborative Research Group Registry. Outcome following thiopurine use in children with UC: a prospective multicenter registry study. *Am J Gastroenterol.* 2011;106(5):981-987.
3. Kotlyar DS, Osterman MT, Diamond RH, et al. A systematic review of factors that contribute to hepatosplenic T-cell lymphoma in patients with inflammatory bowel disease. *Clin Gastroenterol Hepatol.* 2010;9(1):36-41.
4. Turner D, Grossman AB, Rosh J, et al. Methotrexate following unsuccessful thiopurine therapy in pediatric Crohn's disease. *Am J Gastroenterol* 2007;102(12):2804-2812.
5. Hyams J, Crandall W, Kugathasan S, et al; REACH Study Group. Induction and maintenance infliximab therapy for the treatment of moderate-to-severe Crohn's disease in children. *Gastroenterology.* 2007;132(3):863-873.
6. Hyams JS, Griffiths A, Markowitz J, et al. Safety and efficacy of adalimumab for moderate to severe Crohn's disease in children. *Gastroenterology.* 2012;143(2):365-74.e2. doi: 10.1053/j.gastro.2012.04.046. Epub 2012 May 2.

42

HOW DO I KNOW IF MY PATIENT WITH INFLAMMATORY BOWEL DISEASE IS TRULY IN REMISSION AND DOING WELL?

Peter Church, MD and Anne M. Griffiths, MD, FRCPC

Physicians providing general pediatric care to children and adolescents with Crohn's disease and ulcerative colitis (UC) are often called upon to judge whether their patient's inflammatory bowel disease (IBD) is under control or in remission. Although both of these major forms of IBD have traditionally been viewed as disorders with remissions and exacerbations, we now recognize that clinical remission or symptom control is not the same as resolution of intestinal inflammation. Increasingly, pediatric IBD specialists are concerned with healing the diseased intestine in the hopes of preventing long-term complications of Crohn's disease and UC.

Clinical Remission: Symptoms and Growth

For a long time, children with IBD were felt to be in remission if they did not complain of any symptoms and continued to grow in height and gain weight appropriately and develop normally. This is called *clinical remission* and can be thought of as the minimum requirement for establishing that your patient with IBD is doing well.

However, assessing remission just based on symptoms can be misleading. For example, children accustomed to living with chronically active Crohn's inflammation are known to under-report abdominal pain because they are so accustomed to it, so you need to pay close attention to their rate of growth and also to additional markers of inflammation. Active UC is almost invariably associated with visible blood, but urgent, loose nonbloody stools in a teenaged patient with definite chronic UC are more likely due to infection or irritable bowel syndrome. Hence, it is possible to both underestimate and overestimate the activity of IBD by relying only on reported clinical symptoms.

Normal growth is a marker of therapy success in IBD and can provide a very important objective marker of the status of inflammation in the intestine. You should measure height and weight regularly, and assess your patient's rate of growth (height velocity), taking into account what you expect for his or her pubertal stage. Identifying abnormal growth requires a good understanding of the range of normal growth patterns during childhood and adolescence. A decrease in height velocity is very common prior to the diagnosis of Crohn's disease. Likewise, a continued slow rate of linear growth is an important clinical indicator of undertreated Crohn's disease after diagnosis. We cannot overemphasize the importance of measuring height regularly. We now know that the most important factor responsible for impaired growth in chronic inflammatory conditions is the direct effect of proinflammatory cytokines on growing bone. The best way to ensure adequate linear growth in your patients with Crohn's disease is to eliminate inflammation, but without the need for chronic daily steroid therapy. In UC, impaired linear growth is much less common, but children should still be monitored.

Clinical Activity Indices

Multi-item measures or disease activity indices have been developed and validated as means of judging the degree of active inflammation. The Pediatric Crohn's Disease Activity Index (PCDAI) and the Pediatric Ulcerative Colitis Activity Index (PUCAI) incorporate the items most important in reflecting disease activity in Crohn's disease and UC, respectively. They are more objective and reproducible than a simple gut feeling.

PEDIATRIC CROHN'S DISEASE ACTIVITY INDEX

The PCDAI combines abdominal pain, number of stools per day, general well-being, hematocrit, erythrocyte sedimentation rate (ESR), albumin, weight, height velocity, abdominal tenderness, perirectal disease, and extra-intestinal manifestations with a range of scores from 0 to 100. It has been reworked several times over the years into abbreviated forms, and most recently has been reweighted mathematically (wPCDAI)[1] with a value <12.5 indicating remission. This newest index performs better in assessing patients and is more feasible.

PEDIATRIC ULCERATIVE COLITIS ACTIVITY INDEX

The PUCAI[2] combines ratings of abdominal pain, rectal bleeding, stool consistency, number of stools per day, presence of nocturnal stools, and overall activity level (Table 42-1). Most importantly, if you use this index in assessing your UC patients, you should be able to recognize those with severe disease (PUCAI in the range of 65 or greater) who will need urgent hospitalization and intravenous steroid treatment.

Beyond Symptoms: Deep Remission

As we move forward, our therapeutic targets in IBD are moving beyond simple clinical remission and symptom control to *deep remission*, which is actual healing of the intestinal mucosa and surrounding tissues. There has been convincing evidence, as would be expected, that if complete healing of the mucosa is achieved, there are better long-term outcomes.

Table 42-1
The Pediatric Ulcerative Colitis Activity Index

Item	Points
1. Abdominal pain	
No pain	0
Pain can be ignored	5
Pain cannot be ignored	10
2. Rectal bleeding	
None	0
Small amount only, in less than 50% of stools	10
Small amount with most stools	20
Large amount (>50% of the stool content)	30
3. Stool consistency of most stools	
Formed	0
Partially formed	5
Completely unformed	10
4. Number of stools per 24 hours	
0 to 2	0
3 to 5	5
6 to 8	10
>8	15
5. Nocturnal stools (any episode causing wakening)	
No	0
Yes	10
6. Activity level	
No limitation of activity	0
Occasional limitation of activity	5
Severe restricted activity	10
Sum of PUCAI (0 to 85)	
Remission: <10; mild disease: 10 to 30; Moderate disease: 35 to 65; severe disease: >65	

Particularly in Crohn's disease, there is a well recognized disconnect between symptoms reported and the degree of visible inflammation in the bowel. This is demonstrated in Figure 42-1, in which there is no correlation between the Crohn's disease activity index (CDAI) used in adults (which relies very heavily on symptoms) and the appearance of the ileocolon.

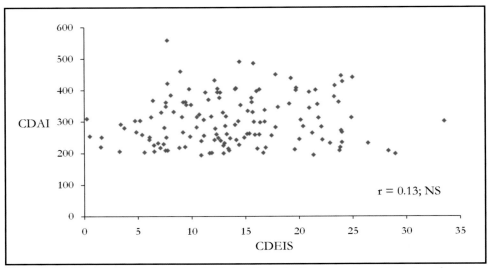

Figure 42-1. No correlation between CDAI and Crohn's disease endoscopic index of severity (CDEIS). (Reprinted with permission from Modigliani R, Mary JY, Simon JF, et al. Clinical, biological, and endoscopic picture of attacks of Crohn's disease. Evolution on prednisolone. Groupe d'Etude Therapeutique des Affections Inflammatoires Digestives. *Gastroenterology.* 1990;98[4]:811-818.)

Repeating a colonoscopy frequently is not practical, and so we look for less-invasive surrogate markers that reflect active mucosal disease better than symptoms. These include blood tests, fecal tests, and imaging. Note that PCDAI incorporates some blood test results.

Serum Biomarkers of Disease Activity

Acute phase proteins are defined as those proteins where the concentrations change by more than 25% during inflammation. They are usually produced by hepatocytes in response to inflammatory cytokines. They all have different kinetic properties and are often discordant. ESR and C-reactive protein (CRP) are nonspecific, meaning they reflect inflammation anywhere. Another inflammatory marker, alpha-1-acid glycoprotein/orosomucoid (a1AGP), is thought to be more specific to bowel inflammation. Serum albumin and platelet count will also change with inflammatory activity in some patients.

Each patient tends to have an inflammatory fingerprint, so that for each flare, the same set of markers tend to become abnormal.[4] For example, if your patient is known to have an elevated CRP but not ESR during disease flares, you should monitor the CRP and pay less attention to the ESR.

C-Reactive Protein

CRP binds phosphocholine expressed on cell surfaces and helps to activate the complement system. It is released from the liver in response to inflammatory cytokines. Older studies have shown that CRP is elevated in nearly 100% of patients with Crohn's disease and about 50% of patients with UC. The most recent review showed that CRP correlates with endoscopic disease with a coefficient of only about 0.45 to 0.6.[5] On the other hand, if your patient has active symptoms and an elevated CRP, the likelihood that he or she has active mucosal disease is very high. You must remember that active mucosal disease can be present in either Crohn's disease or UC even if the CRP is normal.

Erythrocyte Sedimentation Rate

ESR is the rate at which erythrocytes settle when blood is placed in an upright (Westergren) tube. This rate is governed by the balance of factors that speed-up and slow-down the fall of erythrocytes. The largest contributor to erythrocytes clumping together, and thus falling faster, is increased fibrinogen, another protein released by the liver in response to inflammation. This measure of inflammation is more indirect than CRP and can be confounded by changes in red blood cell size. Similar to CRP, ESR tends to be increased more commonly in patients with Crohn's disease than in UC, but ESR changes more slowly than CRP.

FECAL BIOMARKERS

Since the performance of serum biomarkers in reflecting intestinal inflammation is so imperfect, fecal biomarkers have been developed and are regularly used by physicians in Europe in monitoring their young IBD patients.

Calprotectin is a protein that binds calcium and zinc. It is the most common protein found in granulocyte cytoplasm, and thus its presence in stool indicates a neutrophilic infiltrate. Lactoferrin is an iron-binding protein that is similarly present within neutrophils, but it is also formed in the serum and is secreted by mucosal surfaces. Both calprotectin and lactoferrin are resistant to degradation and are stable at room temperature for several days. Fecal calprotectin and lactoferrin have sensitivities and specificities for detection of mucosal inflammation of greater than 80%.[5] Calprotectin has been shown to correlate well with active endoscopic disease, and lactoferrin is quite similar.[5] Both fecal tests are better at detecting activity in the colon than in the ileum and many studies have shown that future relapse of UC (and Crohn's disease to a lesser extent) is predicted by elevation in fecal calprotectin. Hopefully these fecal inflammatory markers will be accessible to patients in North America in the near future, as there is general consensus that they are superior to serum markers in reflecting intestinal inflammation.

IMAGING

The main imaging modalities useful in the assessment of patients with IBD are ultrasound (US), computed tomography enterography (CTE), and magnetic resonance enterography (MRE). A high correlation exists between presence of lesions detected on US, CTE, or MRE and changes seen at endoscopy. Unsurprisingly, poor correlation is found between changes on US, CTE, or MRE and clinical activity indices.[6] Since the performances of all 3 technologies are similar, the choice of modality comes down to other factors. The main drawbacks of US are that it is so highly operator dependent, time consuming, difficult to standardize, and challenging to archive for comparison with subsequent studies. Additionally, not all bowel loops are always accessible by US, especially in larger patients. CTE is very sensitive and specific for inflammatory changes in the bowel, but the large risk from ionizing radiation means it should not be used in children. Thus, it is MRE that is emerging as the favorite imaging modality for the assessment of pediatric IBD, since it is just as sensitive and specific as the other 2 modalities, eliminates the risk of ionizing radiation, is standardized, and is easily reproducible. Imaging technologies have now advanced to eliminate the motion artefact that hampered early MR studies of the bowel. In our practice, MRE is useful for routine reassessment of the entire gastrointestinal tract, but especially the small bowel, as it is best distended by the oral contrast and cannot be completely assessed by colonoscopy.

Conclusion

Minimum criteria for defining remission today for a patient with IBD include normal patterns of development and growth (height, weight, and height velocity) and absence of symptoms. However, symptoms alone can be inadequate and misleading. Thus, treating IBD today requires moving beyond symptom control. Following serum and fecal biomarkers of inflammation combined with periodic imaging with MRE will allow us to move toward the goal of attaining deep remission (that is absence of symptoms and a healed intestine) for all our patients with IBD.

References

1. Turner D, Griffiths AM, Walters TD, et al. Mathematical weighting of the pediatric Crohn's disease activity index (PCrohn's diseaseAI) and comparison with its other short versions. *Inflamm Bowel Dis.* 2012;18(1):55-62.
2. Turner D, Otley AR, Mack D, et al. Development, validation, and evaluation of a pediatric UC activity index: a prospective multicenter study. *Gastroenterology.* 2007;133(2):423-432.
3. Modigliani R, Mary JY, Simon JF, et al. Clinical, biological, and endoscopic picture of attacks of Crohn's disease. Evolution on prednisolone. Groupe d'Etude Therapeutique des Affections Inflammatoires Digestives. *Gastroenterology.* 1990;98(4):811-818.
4. Turner D, Mack DR, Hyams J, et al. C-reactive protein (CRP), erythrocyte sedimentation rate (ESR) or both? A systematic evaluation in pediatric UC. *J Crohns Colitis.* 2011;5(5):423-429.
5. Lewis JD. The utility of biomarkers in the diagnosis and therapy of inflammatory bowel disease. *Gastroenterology.* 2011;140(6):1817-1826.
6. Panes J, Bouzas R, Chaparro M, et al. Systematic review: the use of ultrasonography, computed tomography and magnetic resonance imaging for the diagnosis, assessment of activity and abdominal complications of Crohn's disease. *Aliment Pharmacol Ther.* 2011;34(2):125-145.

43

What Routine Health Maintenance Is Needed for the Pediatric Inflammatory Bowel Disease Patient?

Emily R. Perito, MD, MAS and Melvin B. Heyman, MD, MPH

Approximately 25% of patients with Crohn's disease or ulcerative colitis (UC) present before the age of 18.[1] After a child or adolescent is diagnosed with inflammatory bowel disease (IBD), the general pediatrician retains an important role in that child's care.

Monitoring Growth and Nutritional Status

Growth and nutrition are important markers of disease activity and outcome in children with IBD. Many "fall off their curves" with slowed velocities of weight gain and/or linear growth prior to diagnosis. In fact, weight loss and a slowing of growth velocity can be the earliest symptoms of IBD, even before the development of gastrointestinal (GI) symptoms. Following diagnosis, ongoing assessment of growth is crucial to help children reach their growth potential and to detect persistently active disease.

Evaluating the child's growth curve at each health care visit is essential. If a child has become underweight or has slowed growth velocity prior to IBD diagnosis, we expect to see catch-up growth in the months following treatment initiation. A child's prior growth velocity and mid-parental height can be used to assess whether children with IBD are on the appropriate growth curve. Delayed bone age is common in children with IBD; evaluation with wrist radiographs for bone age can help predict remaining growth potential.[1]

Unintentional declines in weight or body mass index (BMI) or an unexpected slowing of height velocity can be a sign of active IBD. If such changes are noted, the child should be assessed for active IBD in consultation with a pediatric gastroenterologist. Celiac disease (CD) and thyroid disease should also be considered.

Children with IBD are at risk for inadequate nutrition and vitamin deficiencies. We recommend evaluating nutritional status with a complete blood cell count, iron studies (iron, ferritin, and total iron binding capacity), 25-OH vitamin D, folate, vitamin B_{12}, zinc levels, and prothrombin time (as a marker of vitamin-K status) at diagnosis and at routine intervals. Some centers recommend annual assessment, while others evaluate depending on disease location and activity. For example, prior to diagnosis and with disease flares, children can develop iron deficiency secondary to ongoing GI blood loss. In children with Crohn's disease, inflammation in the terminal ileum can lead to malabsorption of fat-soluble vitamins and vitamin B_{12}. Zinc levels can be helpful in children with persistent poor growth or diarrhea despite controlled IBD.

IBD carries an increased risk of osteopenia because of chronic nutritional deficiencies and possibly because of the chronic inflammation. A dual-energy x-ray absorptiometry (DEXA) scan to evaluate bone mineral density (BMD) is recommended at IBD diagnosis. When interpreting DEXA in children, it is important to use z-scores that compare a child's BMD to age and sex-matched peers, rather than t-scores that use lifetime peak BMD as a reference. Z-scores < −1 are considered low and should be managed in conjunction with a pediatric gastroenterologist and endocrinologist. We recommend repeat DEXA in children with previously diagnosed osteopenia and in children who develop osteopenia risk factors, including height, weight, or BMI z-scores < −2, delayed puberty, severe IBD, history of severe or multiple fractures, and 6 months or longer of continuous steroid exposure.[2]

Puberty stage should be assessed at all follow-up visits. Puberty is often delayed in children with IBD because of poor nutritional status and systemic inflammation. Recent menses history should be elicited in girls.[1] Secondary amenorrhea is a red flag for IBD diagnosis or disease flares. If an adolescent female's period becomes irregular or stops, assess for disease activity in consultation with a pediatric gastroenterologist.

Vaccinations

Children and adolescents with IBD are at an increased risk of infections due to underlying chronic disease and immunosuppressive therapy. Appropriate vaccination is essential to protect these children from preventable infections. Attention to the type of vaccine and the child's immunosuppressive medication is crucial for safe and effective vaccination.

Children with IBD should receive nonlive vaccines on the regular immunization schedule[3] (Table 43-1). Delays might be considered while a child is on high-dose systemic steroids (>2 mg/kg/day or >20 mg/day) because of decreased response to the vaccine. But delays are not recommended while a child is on other maintenance immunosuppressive medication, as these are usually continued indefinitely to maintain remission.

Children on high-dose maintenance immunosuppression should not receive live or attenuated vaccines (see Table 43-1). Healthy-close contacts of immunosuppressed children with IBD can receive live vaccines safely.[3] Specific Centers for Disease Control (CDC) guidelines for nonroutine, travel-related vaccines should be consulted prior to administration.[3]

It is particularly important to make sure that older children and adolescents with IBD are up-to-date on their vaccines, as their visits to the pediatrician are less frequent. Make sure to give these patients tetanus-diphtheria-pertussis (TdaP), human papillomavirus (HPV), and meningococcal vaccines when age appropriate. One dose of 13-valent pneumococcal conjugate vaccine (PCV13) should be given to children with IBD between 6 and 18 years of age. An injectable flu vaccine should be given annually.[3]

IBD patients have an increased risk of getting HPV, and those with Crohn's disease have an increased risk of developing perianal cancer. Women with IBD have an increased likelihood of abnormal pap smears as adults.[4] Thus, the HPV vaccine is important in males and females with IBD.

Patients with IBD are thought to mount normal response to vaccines, but treatments, including immunosuppressive and anti-tumor necrosis factor (anti-TNF) medications, may blunt this.

Table 43-1

Recommendations for Vaccination in Children with Inflammatory Bowel Disease

Vaccine Type	Specific Vaccines	Recommendations in IBD
Live and attenuated vaccines	Viral: Intranasal influenza MMR *Varicella* Zoster Rotavirus Yellow fever Vaccinia (smallpox) Bacterial: Oral typhoid vaccine BCG	Contraindicated in children on systemic corticosteroids >2 mg/kg/day or >20 mg/day for children >10 kg; defer for at least 1 month after stopping systemic steroid
		Contraindicated in children receiving monoclonal antibody therapies (eg, infliximab, certolizumab, or adalimumab)
		Contraindicated in children on chronic immunosuppressive medications (eg, 6-mercaptopurine, azathioprine, or methotrexate)
		Household or other close contacts of children on these immunosuppressive medications can safely receive live virus vaccines
Inactivated vaccines	DTaP/Tdap Hib IPV Intramuscular influenza Hepatitis A Hepatitis B Meningococcal PCV13 HPV	Safe and recommended on age-appropriate schedule
		Annual injectable influenza vaccine recommended
		One dose of PCV13 recommended between 6 to 18 years of age

MMR: measles, mumps, and rubella; BCG: bacille Calmette-Guérin; Hib: Haemophilus influenzae type B; IPV: inactivated poliovirus; PCV13: Pneumococcal; HPV: human papilloma virus.

Checking vaccine titers can help with the assessment of immunization status and response to vaccines in children with IBD; however, this is not recommended as part of routine care.

Screening for latent tuberculosis (TB) with a tuberculin skin test (TST) should be done on a routine schedule for IBD patients and should be repeated immediately prior to starting anti-TNF therapy (eg, infliximab, adalimumab, or certolizumab). Any TST with 5 mm or greater diameter of induration is considered positive in an immunosuppressed patient.[4] Nonresponse to the TST

Table 43-2

Extra-Intestinal Manifestations of Inflammatory Bowel Disease in Children and Adolescents

- Growth failure with weight loss and short stature
- Anemia
- Eyes: uveitis, iritis, glaucoma, retinal vasculitis, optical neuritis
- Oropharynx: aphthous ulcers, aphthous stomatitis
- GI: perianal skin tags or fistulas, pancreatitis
- Liver: primary sclerosing cholangitis, autoimmune hepatitis
- Renal: kidney stones
- Endocrine: amenorrhea (eg, primary or secondary)
- Joints: arthritis, arthralgias, ankylosing spondylitis
- Skin: erythema nodosum, pyoderma gangrenosum, psoriasis
- Bone: osteopenia/osteoporosis, compression fractures

(anergy) in patients on immunosuppressive agents is a possibility; in children with high suspicion for TB, control skin tests with candida, tetanus, or mumps can be considered. Anti-TNF therapy carries a risk of reactivation of latent tuberculosis, and in those with a positive-skin test or chest radiograph, initiation of therapy with isoniazid or another regimen is recommended before the anti-TNF medication is started.

Hepatitis B surface antigen (indicative of active infection) and surface antibody (indicative of protective immunity) tests should also be done prior to initiating anti-TNF therapy. Active hepatitis B infection is a contraindication to anti-TNF therapy.[4] While hepatitis B is relatively uncommon in children, it is usually an asymptomatic disease in this age group so screening is important.

Screening for Extra-Intestinal Manifestations of Inflammatory Bowel Disease

Ongoing monitoring for the development of extra-intestinal manifestations of IBD should occur at all visits (Table 43-2). Approximately 30% of all children diagnosed with IBD develop extra-intestinal manifestations. Arthritis and oral aphthous ulcers affect 20% to 25% of children with IBD after diagnosis.[5] Common skin manifestations include erythema nodosum (painful red nodules, usually on the shins), pyoderma gangrenosum (chronic ulcers, usually on the legs or at sites of prior trauma), and psoriasis. All patients with IBD should have an annual ophthalmologic exam to evaluate for uveitis, iritis, or glaucoma as a manifestation of IBD and for glaucoma or cataracts as an adverse effect of prolonged corticosteroid therapy. Symptomatic extra-intestinal manifestations are signs of active systemic inflammation and often respond to adjustments or additions to a child's treatment regimen aimed at intestinal inflammation.

Psychological Well-Being in Inflammatory Bowel Disease

IBD and its complications can put considerable stress on children and their families. Concerns about their chronic medical condition and medications, stress caused by interruptions to school or other activities, and physical symptoms of IBD can lead to depression and anxiety in both children and parents.[6] Routine screening for these conditions in both children and caregivers should also occur at all primary care visits.

Depression and anxiety can increase the risk for noncompliance with IBD treatments, which can lead to disease flares, complications, and sometimes worsening psychological distress. Irritable bowel syndrome and other functional GI disorders can coexist with IBD and have symptoms exacerbated by stress, depression, and anxiety. Psychological comorbidities do not necessarily correlate with IBD activity or severity but can substantially impact a patient's quality of life.[6] Differentiating functional symptoms from active IBD can be difficult and should be undertaken in partnership with the pediatric gastroenterologist.

Although children and adolescents with IBD should see their pediatric gastroenterologist every 3 to 6 months, routine health maintenance with their pediatrician is also crucial. Adequate routine health care is important to ensure that children with IBD achieve their growth potential, are adequately protected by vaccines, and have their extra-intestinal manifestations appropriately diagnosed and controlled.

References

1. Heuschkel R, Salvestrini C, Beattie RM, Hildebrand H, Walters T, Griffiths A. Guidelines for the management of growth failure in childhood inflammatory bowel disease. *Inflamm Bowel Dis.* 2008;14(6):839–849.
2. Pappa H, Thayu M, Sylvester F, Leonard M, Zemel B, Gordon C. Skeletal health of children and adolescents with inflammatory bowel disease. *J Pediatr Gastrenterol Nutr.* 2011;53:11-25.
3. Kroger AT, Sumaya CV, Pickering LK, Atkinson WL. General recommendations on immunization: Recommendations of the Advisory Committee on Immunization Practices. *MMWR.* 2011;60(2):3-61.
4. Moscandrew M, Mahadevan U, Kane S. General health maintenance in IBD. *Inflamm Bowel Dis.* 2009;15(9): 1399-1409.
5. Jose FA, Garnett EA, Vittinghoff E, et al. Development of extraintestinal manifestations in pediatric patients with inflammatory bowel disease. *Inflamm Bowel Dis.* 2009;15(1):63-68.
6. Karwowski CA, Keljo D, Szigethy E. Strategies to improve quality of life in adolescents with inflammatory bowel disease. *Inflamm Bowel Dis.* 2009;15(11):1755-1764.

HOW CAN I FACILITATE THE TRANSITION OF MY ADOLESCENT PATIENT WITH INFLAMMATORY BOWEL DISEASE TO THE ADULT HEALTH CARE TEAM?

Namita Singh, MD and Marla Dubinsky, MD

Inflammatory bowel disease (IBD) is diagnosed before the age of 18 years in up to 25% of patients. Given that the disease is often chronic and can be more aggressive in patients diagnosed at a younger age, the transition from pediatric to adult care is of high importance. For a healthy adolescent, the years of transition to adulthood are marked by significant changes and new challenges. For chronically ill adolescents, this complex period is compounded by the burden of having a disease. The goal of transition to adult health care is to achieve a continuum of care with the acquisition of independent skills, along with personal development. This transition process remains a challenge involving the patient, patient's family, and health care team.

In the North American Society for Pediatric Gastroenterology, Hepatology, and Nutrition (NASPGHAN) statement[1] regarding pediatric IBD, the recommendations are to start the process of transition by taking the following 4 steps:

1. Seeing adolescents without their parents.

2. Discussing with the patient and family the benefits of transition to an adult gastroenterology practice.

3. Developing a relationship with an adult gastroenterologist who is knowledgeable in caring for young adults with childhood-onset IBD.

4. Providing all of the necessary medical records and summaries so the family will realize that all providers are working together to deliver excellent care.

To initiate this process, the pediatric gastroenterologist should sit down with the patient and family to discuss the need and timing for a smooth transition. The benefits should be expressed, including the normalization of development, promotion of independent behavior, improvement of compliance with therapy, provision of an appropriate environment, and formation of long-term goals. The pediatric gastroenterologist should encourage visits without parents to build a relationship that promotes self-reliance and resembles the relationship they will have with their adult gastroenterologist.

During this time, if not prior, adolescent patients should become fully educated on IBD, in order to be able to assume personal responsibility for their medical care. This is often difficult, as shown in one study[2] in which adult gastroenterologists were surveyed in regard to the transition-of-care from their pediatric counterparts. Key elements of weakness were recognized; 55% reported that young adults with IBD have deficits in knowledge of their medical condition and 69% reported that the patients had a lack of understanding of their medication regimens. Prior to transferring care, resources and education should be provided, and patients should be encouraged to ask questions and take notes about their disease, procedural history, and medications.

Timing of the transition process is of paramount importance and requires flexibility. The American Academy of Pediatrics recognizes that the timing of transition to adult-oriented health care is unique to each patient and ideally occurs between 18 to 21 years of age. For example, it is recommended that a pediatric gastroenterologist continues to follow adolescents who have additional growth potential, resulting from delayed puberty. Ideally, the transition should occur during a period of disease remission, as to minimize treatment changes during this time. The personal developmental stage of the patient should be assessed to determine the ideal timing for transition. Tools to assess the readiness for transition are available, such as the Transition Readiness Assessment Questionnaire,[3] a validated survey that is used to assess a patient's skills for self-management of chronic conditions, self-advocacy, and the health care utilization.

Once it has been decided to pursue the transition to an adult gastroenterologist, the next step is to identify a skilled gastroenterologist who cares for young adults, recognizes the various differences in childhood-onset IBD, and understands the development of young adults. This may, itself, pose a challenge, as only 46% of adult gastroenterologists reported being competent in areas of young adult and adolescent medicine. Many important issues become more relevant around the time of transition and include sexual health and fertility, as pregnancy carries a higher risk in IBD patients. Substance use and abuse becomes more of an issue during adolescence and young adulthood, and thus it is important that the risks of smoking, alcohol, and drug use are communicated clearly with these patients. Cancer surveillance will also become an important issue to discuss, if it has not occurred already.

Ideally, a joint outpatient visit with both the transferring pediatric physician and the adult gastroenterologist assuming the patient's care will occur. In this visit, the patient is introduced to the new physician and the transferring physician summarizes the patient's disease course and medications verbally with the patient in the room. An open conversation can proceed and a treatment plan outlined with the patient. Given that an overlap period in which there are joint visits with a pediatric and adult gastroenterologist is often not feasible, the transfer of information, including a concise summary of the patient's disease, is important. Of adult gastroenterologists, 51% report receiving inadequate medical history from pediatric providers. It is recommended that a letter summarizing the medical history be sent to the adult gastroenterologist, with a copy given to the patient.

Conclusion

The transition from pediatric to adult IBD health care remains a challenging but fulfilling process. The goals are to facilitate the shift of responsibility from the caregiver to the patient, and to move the patient from a pediatric to adult gastroenterology practice (Figure 44-1). This transition process is often empowering for patients and may reduce noncompliance, as data suggest that autonomy may improve compliance in chronically ill adolescents. Transition is equally

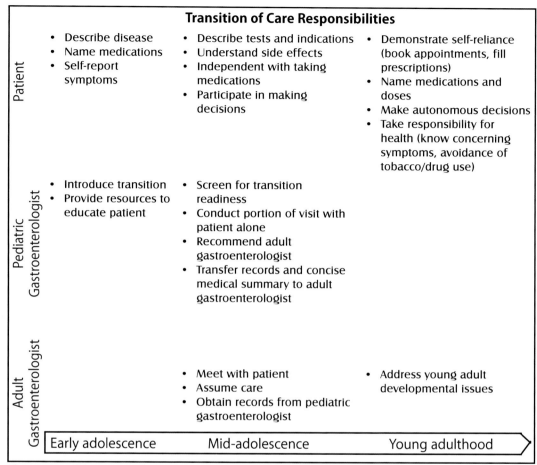

Figure 44-1. Transition of care responsibilities based on the different stages of adolescence and the tasks that should be accomplished by the patient and physicians to facilitate an ideal transition. This is a general guideline; actual transition may vary depending on the patient's maturity, readiness, and other social factors.

important in both academic centers and in private offices, regardless of whether they are full IBD centers or general gastroenterology practices. Successfully transitioned patients are independent and equipped with the resources and knowledge to be as functional, healthy, and well as their disease allows.

References

1. Baldassano R, Ferry G, Griffiths A, Mack D, Markowitz J, Winter H. Transition of the patient with inflammatory bowel disease from pediatric to adult care: recommendations of the North American Society for Pediatric Gastroenterology, Hepatology and Nutrition. *J Pediatr Gastroenterol Nutr.* 2002;34(3):245-248.
2. Hait EJ, Barendse RM, Arnold JH, et al. Transition of adolescents with inflammatory bowel disease from pediatric to adult care: a survey of adult gastroenterologists. *J Pediat Gastroenterol Nutr.* 2009;48(1):61-65.
3. Sawicki GS, Lukens-Bull K, Yin X, et al. Measuring the transition readiness of youth with special healthcare needs: validation of the TRAQ—Transition Readiness Assessment Questionnaire. *J Pediatr Psychol.* 2011;36(2):160-171.

Bibliography

Hait E, Arnold JH, Fishman LN. Educate, communicate, anticipate-practical recommendations for transitioning adolescents with IBD to adult health care. *Inflamm Bowel Dis*. 2006;12(1):70-73.

Philpott JR. Transitional care in inflammatory bowel disease. *Gastroenterol Hepatol* (NY). 2011;7(1):26-32.

45

ARE THERE EMOTIONAL ISSUES THAT ARE COMMONLY SEEN IN PEDIATRIC INFLAMMATORY BOWEL DISEASE THAT I SHOULD LOOK FOR IN MY PATIENTS AND THEIR FAMILIES?

Laura Mackner, PhD and Wallace Crandall, MD

Inflammatory bowel disease (IBD) has the potential to disrupt several areas of emotional adjustment. The disease course is unpredictable, treatment can be frustrating, and the symptoms can be embarrassing and socially limiting. Children with IBD may be reluctant to talk about their symptoms, and their frequent visits to the bathroom can be embarrassing. They may limit their activities to those with ready access to a bathroom, or they may unexpectedly cancel planned activities. The corticosteroid medication often used to treat IBD may impact emotional functioning directly via mood changes and indirectly through appearance-altering side effects. The developmental context should be taken into account, too, since IBD is often diagnosed in adolescence, when rates of emotional problems increase, and social activities and peer acceptance become even more important than earlier in childhood. We will discuss emotional adjustment in the areas of specific symptoms and diagnoses, social, family, and academic functioning, and the overall impact of the disease on typical life activities.

In the area of specific symptoms and diagnoses, rates of current depressive disorders range from 10% to approximately 20%, and a recent meta-analysis reported[1] that youth with IBD are at an increased risk for depressive disorders compared to youth with other chronic illnesses. The rates of current anxiety disorders, which range from 4% in a heterogeneous sample to 28% in a newly diagnosed sample, were not significantly different from youth with other chronic illnesses. When compared to healthy children, the meta-analysis also reported that those with IBD had significantly more internalizing symptoms (anxiety and depression symptoms combined), with up to 31% of children with IBD experiencing clinically significant internalizing symptoms. Table 45-1 shows the primary symptoms of common depressive and anxiety disorders.

Risk factors for developing depression have been investigated and include stressful life events, maternal depression, family dysfunction, and steroid treatment. The role of disease severity is not clear, with an equal number of studies finding a significant or no relationship. While this may seem counter-intuitive, research in other pediatric chronic illnesses has shown that psychosocial

Table 45-1

Primary Symptoms of Depressive and Anxiety Disorders

Major Depressive Disorder

In the past 2 weeks:

- Depressed mood most of the day, nearly every day; in children, can be irritable mood
- Markedly diminished interest or pleasure in almost all activities most of the day, nearly every day
- Significant weight loss when not dieting or weight gain, or decrease or increase in appetite nearly every day; in children, failure to make expected weight gains
- Insomnia or hypersomnia nearly every day
- Psychomotor agitation or retardation nearly every day that is observable by others, not merely subjective feelings
- Feelings of worthlessness or excessive/inappropriate guilt nearly every day
- Diminished ability to think or concentrate, or indecisiveness nearly every day
- Recurrent thoughts of death or suicidal ideation without a plan, or suicide attempt or specific plan for committing suicide

Dysthymic Disorder

In the past year:

- Depressed mood for most of the day, for more days than not; in children and adolescents, mood can be irritable
- Poor appetite or overeating
- Insomnia or hypersomnia
- Low energy or fatigue
- Low self-esteem
- Poor concentration or difficulty making decisions
- Feelings of hopelessness

Generalized Anxiety Disorder

At least 6 months:

- Excessive anxiety and worry about a number of events or activities, occurring more days than not
- Difficulty to controlling the worry
- Restlessness or feeling keyed up or on edge
- Easily fatigued
- Difficulty concentrating or mind going blank
- Irritability
- Muscle tension
- Sleep disturbance (difficulty falling or staying asleep or restless unsatisfying sleep)

(continued)

Table 45-1 (continued)

Primary Symptoms of Depressive and Anxiety Disorders

Social Phobia
At least 6 months: • Marked and persistent fear of a social or performance situation with unfamiliar people or possible scrutiny by others   ◦ Fears will act in a way (or show anxiety symptoms) that will be embarrassing   • Exposure to the feared social situation almost invariably provokes anxiety   • The feared situations are avoided or else endured with intense anxiety or distress
Panic Attack
• Discrete period of intense fear or discomfort; symptoms develop abruptly and reach a peak within 10 minutes   • Palpitations, pounding heart, or accelerated heart rate   • Sweating   • Trembling or shaking   • Sensations of shortness of breath or smothering   • Feeling of choking   • Chest pain or discomfort   • Nausea or abdominal distress   • Dizzy, lightheaded or faint   • Feelings of unreality or being detached from oneself   • Fear of losing control or going crazy   • Fear of dying   • Paresthesias   • Chills or hot flushes

Note: For all disorders, the symptoms must cause clinically significant distress or impairment in important areas of functioning, and the symptoms must not be due to a medical condition or effects of a substance (eg, medication).

factors, such as family-functioning and stress-coping strategies, are better predictors of emotional symptoms than illness factors. For example, a child with good family supports and stress-coping skills may be less likely to develop emotional problems when faced with severe IBD than a child without these resources. Conversely, a child with poor coping skills may have difficulty with emotional issues even when experiencing mild IBD.

In other areas, a meta-analysis reported[1] that youth with IBD have significantly worse social functioning than healthy children,[1] with up to 35% reporting clinically significant social difficulty. Onset of IBD during adolescence increases the risk for social problems, and boys with IBD have more social difficulty than girls (IBD or healthy) and healthy boys.

School functioning presents a mixed picture. Most youth with IBD feel that their condition has negatively affected their grades or educational attainment, but objective data suggest similar levels of academic performance and educational attainment when compared to healthy youth. However, several studies have reported that attendance is significantly worse in those with IBD compared to healthy children, even among those with remitted or mild disease. Children with internalizing symptoms are at increased risk of poor school attendance.[2]

Mixed results have also been reported when examining overall family functioning in those with a child with IBD compared to healthy families. Typically, families report healthy levels of family functioning, but some report difficulty with communication, family roles/responsibilities, and the degree to which family members are involved in one another's lives.[3] Disease severity is associated with family functioning, so this pattern might reflect the course of IBD (ie, remission and flares) and its impact on family life. The demands of IBD may challenge a family's ability to communicate with one another, and family roles/responsibilities may change to accommodate disease flares (eg, one caregiver stays with the ill child in hospital, while the other caregiver cares for healthy children and household tasks). Child emotional symptoms are also associated with family dysfunction.

The overall impact of the disease on one's life is also known as health-related quality of life (QOL). Youth with IBD report similar QOL to that of youth with other chronic and acute medical conditions, and a meta-analysis reported[1] that their QOL is significantly worse when compared to healthy children. Worse disease severity and fatigue increase the risk of lower QOL.

Since youth with IBD are at risk for emotional problems in several areas, these issues should be assessed during a clinic or office visit. Symptoms of depression and anxiety should be assessed (see Table 45-1), as well as QOL and social functioning in multiple areas (eg, social withdrawal, interpersonal difficulty with peers, and difficulty participating in social or athletic activities). School attendance should be assessed, especially among those with internalizing symptoms. Assessing family communication, roles/responsibilities, and the degree to which family members are involved in one another's lives may be useful during disease flares.

In general, it is important for the medical team to differentiate short-term, situational distress related to flares or diagnosis of IBD from more severe symptoms or extended period of impaired functioning when referral may be warranted. If the difficulty significantly affects a child's life and/ or causes significant distress, referral to a mental health professional with training in understanding the unique impact of pediatric chronic illness may be warranted. Cognitive behavioral therapy (CBT) has been shown to be effective in improving depression symptoms, social functioning, and QOL among youth with IBD. Strategies for managing internalizing symptoms related to school absence have not been evaluated in pediatric IBD, but CBT has been effective in healthy children. A 504 plan for "Other Health Impairment" may also be helpful in increasing attendance by allowing unrestricted bathroom access and accommodations for absences so that returning to school does not feel overwhelming for the child.

References

1. Greenley RN, Hommel KA, Nebel J, et al. A meta-analytic review of the psychosocial adjustment of youth with inflammatory bowel disease. *J Pediatr Psychol*. 2010;35(8):857-869.
2. Mackner L, Bickmeier R, Crandall W. School achievement, absence and quality of life in pediatric inflammatory bowel disease. *J Dev Behav Pediatr*. 2012;33(2):106-111.
3. Herzer M, Denson LA, Baldassano RN, Hommel KA. Family functioning and health-related quality of life in adolescents with pediatric inflammatory bowel disease. *Eur J Gastroenterol Hepatol*. 2011;23(1):95-100.

WHAT DO WE KNOW ABOUT ADHERENCE IN INFLAMMATORY BOWEL DISEASE AND ANY CHRONIC PEDIATRIC MEDICAL CONDITION? WHAT CAN I DO TO HELP?

Neal S. LeLeiko, MD, PhD and Debra Lobato, PhD

Sadly, we know that a lot of kids do not take their medicines. We know that the least reliable way to find out if a patient is taking his or her medicines is to ask the patient; asking the parents is not much better. Self-reporting is just not reliable, no matter how good a rapport we might think we have with a patient. There are many different ways to measure adherence. Some studies look at the frequency and timing of medication refills, while others count pills. We have looked at these methods and, at the same time, used electronic pill bottles that note when the medication bottle is opened.[1] Figure 46-1 shows what these pill bottles look like. The tops of the bottles contain a microchip that records the date and time when it is opened. The bottles are expensive to purchase and require a research assistant to regularly check in to make certain that they are being used correctly. That probably explains why they have not been used very much. Also, everyone is regularly reminded that their adherence is being checked, so that might affect results.

Even though the electronic bottles we use probably serve as reminders, we have found that kids simply do not open their medication bottles as often as we prescribe or as often as we would guess that they do. Furthermore, even clinicians, who know research is being conducted and are attuned to the issue of adherence, are unable to accurately predict who their nonadherent patients are.

On average, kids with inflammatory bowel disease (IBD) and other chronic conditions generally open their pill bottles about half of the time that they are supposed to. It is astonishing that about one-third of our patients open their pill about one-third of the times we would expect. We can only assume that they are taking all of the meds we have prescribed when they do open the bottle. It is a reasonable guess that they are taking the dose of 6-MP we have prescribed, which is usually a whole or fraction of a pill, but unlikely that they are taking all of the 5-ASA tabs prescribed, since this is often many pills at one time.

It is not surprising that the lowest levels of adherence occur in the older adolescents. It is disconcerting that in the younger children, those where we expect the parents to control medication, adherence measured by these electronic pill caps is still far from acceptable. Note that most studies

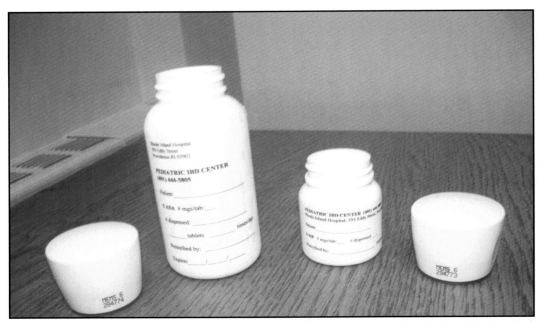

Figure 46-1. Pill bottles used in our studies to determine if patients are opening their medication. Each top is fitted with a microchip that records the time of opening.

cite acceptable adherence to be 80% or better. We really have no data to inform us what level of adherence is actually necessary for clinical response in IBD. Reported rates of adherence in IBD are similar to rates of adherence in other populations with chronic diseases, including diabetes[2] and asthma.[3] However, a majority of the results on adherence in IBD are based on self-report with adherence rates around 80.[4] When more objective methods of adherence are used, such as pill-counts, refill-counts, and 6TGN-assays, adherence rates drop to about 50%.[5]

These low levels of adherence occur in educated, economically comfortable families but are probably worse in children from disadvantaged families. None of the results of adherence studies among children with IBD contradict anything that has been reported among children with other chronic illnesses, such as asthma.

We have noted several different patterns of adherence. Some children just do not take their medications at all. Some take them much more when they are symptomatic and less when they are well. Some take them very regularly for their illness, but barely take them for postsurgical prophylaxis. For some, there is no pattern.

To date, we do not understand enough about why the medicine is not taken. Studies suggest that worse adherence is associated with children (and their parents) who report more behavioral problems and depressive symptoms, such as feeling irritable or sad. This does not mean that you (or any pediatric gastroenterologist) can tell that a child is depressed, and therefore not taking his or her medications. It does mean that compared to peers with better adherence, the children with poor adherence (and their parents) are apt to acknowledge more symptoms associated with depression (but not diagnostic of clinical depression).

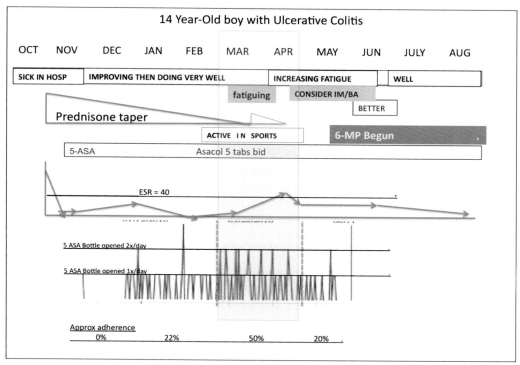

Figure 46-2. Clinical course of a 14-year-old boy with UC demonstrating step-up therapy to 6-mercaptopurine, following a period of nonadherence to 5-ASA. Physician notes indicate a consideration of immunomodulator or biologic agent (IM/BA) at the time that fatigue is noted. By mid-May, 6-MP has begun, and within 2 weeks, the patient reports feeling better and ESR has improved. Of note, the patient doubled the adherence to 5-ASA in the 2 months prior to his improvement, and it is generally agreed that improvement with 6-MP should not be expected before 10 to 12 weeks of therapy. The key question here is: If you were this child's parent, and you knew that he was barely taking his medications, would you have stepped-up to 6-MP at that time, or would you have made sure he was taking his medication?

We think it is very important that if a child is not responding to the medication you have prescribed, you consider in your differential diagnosis the strong possibility that the medication is not being taken in the way you expect. Figure 46-2 illustrates the clinical course of a 14-year-old boy with ulcerative colitis (UC) over time. The case serves to demonstrate 2 underappreciated aspects of poor adherence. First, since the child is not taking his medications regularly, one potential option would have been to increase the dose of his medicine. This could produce significant toxicity. We have heard anecdotes from several colleagues about cases, such as this where dose escalation of 6-mercaptourine led to hepatotoxicity. Only later were caretakers to learn that the medication was being discarded instead of ingested. The second aspect is represented by what actually did occur with this patient. The physicians in charge assumed that this was a medication failure and stepped-up therapy to an immunomodulator. We have no way of knowing what the outcome might have been had the child been adherent to his 5-ASA as prescribed.

Conclusion

We believe that it might be helpful to involve a child psychologist with all pediatric IBD patients and especially those who are not doing well. If one is not available in a family-centered care approach, then we would consider referral of a child who is not doing as well as expected to a child psychologist to help identify characteristics of the child, the family, or the environment that may be interfering with the child's adherence. Behavioral health interventions can help families discover and alter their beliefs and attitudes about their illness and medications, can target children's depressive and behavioral symptoms, and can help families organize routines and strategies for monitoring and encouraging adherence.

Some researchers are looking at the use of special electronic devices and various smart phone applications to assess adherence, as well as to remind children to take their medications. The problem with these devices is that they represent an electronic means of self-reporting, and as such we suspect they may be no more reliable. As far as using them for reminding the patients, this may work or may be an oversimplification of the nature of the problem.

The question of nonadherence to medication is very vexing and probably very complex. It likely will require different solutions for different patients. It is, however, a problem that we all must confront.

References

1. Lobato D, McQuaid E, Nassau J, et al. Rates and predictors of oral medication adherence in pediatric IBD. *Gastroenterology.* 2011;140(supp 1):S91.
2. Odegard PS, Capoccia K. Medication taking and diabetes: a systematic review of the literature. *Diabetes Educ.* 2007;33(6):1014-1029.
3. Pando S, Lemière C, Beauchesne MF, Perreault S, Forget A, Blais L. Suboptimal use of inhaled corticosteroids in children with persistent asthma: inadequate prescription, poor drug adherence, or both? *Pharmacotherapy.* 2010;30(11):1109-1116.
4. Bernal I, Domenech E, Garcia-Planella E, et al. Medication-taking behavior in a cohort of patients with inflammatory bowel disease. *Dig Dis Sci.* 2006;51(12):2165-2169.
5. Hommel KA, Davis CM, Baldassano RN. Objective versus subjective assessment of oral medication adherence in pediatric inflammatory bowel disease. *Inflamm Bowel Dis.* 2009;15(4):589-593.

SECTION IX

PEDIATRIC GASTROINTESTINAL ENDOSCOPY

47

HOW SHOULD I COUNSEL PATIENTS AND FAMILIES REGARDING SCREENING COLONOSCOPY WHEN THERE IS A FAMILY HISTORY OF EARLY COLORECTAL CANCER?

Leigha Senter, MS, CGC and Steven H. Erdman, MD

Colon cancer is thought to have a hereditary component in up to a third of cases and is often suggested when there are 2 or more affected family members or presentation before age 50. Yet, at what age an inherited risk is expressed as an identifiable cancer or precancerous lesion varies greatly, even within the same family. Children, adolescents, and even young adults may be too young to have precancerous polyps, so performing a colonoscopy as a screening test may not rule out the presence of an inherited colon cancer syndrome. Being both invasive and expensive, a colonoscopy should have clear indications.

If Screening Does Not Start With Colonoscopy as the First Step, Provided the Child or Young Adult Has No Digestive Symptoms, Where Should the Evaluation Begin?

Some families with hereditary risks for colon cancer will have well-defined syndromes that are associated with increased risks of both gastrointestinal (GI) and extra-intestinal cancers, such as Lynch syndrome (LS), familial adenomatous polyposis (FAP), *MUTYH*-associated polyposis, Peutz-Jegher syndrome, and juvenile polyposis syndrome. Some—but not all—of these syndromes would warrant endoscopic screening based on age and symptoms as supported by published guidelines and the family history. For this reason, it is important to determine, when possible, the hereditary condition present in the family. Knowing the syndrome will greatly help to determine each individual family members' management plan, but this is not always feasible.

In our opinion, optimal evaluation of the patient and family is a team effort that uses the expertise of many specialists, including those of a genetic counselor specializing in cancer genetics. The genetic counselor will retrieve and review the medical records of those in the family with colon cancer and other key diagnoses and will construct a pedigree by asking questions about cancer histories and colonoscopies in at least 3 generations of your patient's family. Based on this risk assessment, the genetics team will work with the family to determine the best plan of action for genetic testing. In most cases, it is beneficial to begin genetic testing in a family with a person who has a confirmed diagnosis associated with the hereditary syndrome (usually colon cancer or polyps with confirmed histology). Regardless of the outcome of genetic counseling and testing in your patient's family, the genetics team should follow up with you regarding recommendations for your patient and his or her family and will work with you as part of the patient's care team.

In some of the syndromes mentioned, such as in FAP, a screening colonoscopy (to identify if the polyps are present) is recommended to start in childhood. Based on updated guidelines for FAP from the National Comprehensive Cancer Network (www.nccn.org), the initial screening colonoscopy should take place between 10 to 15 years of age. For FAP, once adenomatous polyps are identified, a surveillance colonoscopy should take place yearly to monitor for disease progression. It is important to remember that even within these well-described syndromes, the age at which precancerous polyps develop can vary greatly within and between families.

Where Can I Find a Genetic Counselor? Can This Be Done Over the Internet?

Genetic counselors are available in most metropolitan areas. You can search for a genetic counselor specializing in hereditary cancer through the National Society of Genetic Counselors Web site (www.nsgc.org). In addition to finding genetics services near your patient's home, genetic counseling services are available through multiple phone and Internet services (InformedDNA, for instance, at www.informeddna.com). This is helpful in remote areas where a genetic counselor may be more difficult to reach.

As the Primary Care Provider, Should I Order Genetic Testing as Suggested in All of Those Advertisements?

Technically, any physician can order genetic testing; however, it is helpful to include a genetic counselor in the process. At times, it can be difficult to know which laboratory to choose when ordering a specific genetic screening test, and it often comes down to methodology offered and billing processes. As part of your team, a genetic counselor will also be able to help interpret genetic test results that, at times, provide less-than-clear results—either a genetic variant of uncertain significance or a negative result in a seemingly classically affected individual. It is nice to have an established relationship for collaboration on these cases, and you can work with the genetics team to devise a personalized cancer screening plan for your patient and family based on medical history and genetic test results.

Other Than Early Colorectal Cancer, What Other Family History Findings Suggest a Cancer Syndrome That Should Be Evaluated?

In the past 20 years, much has been learned about inherited cancer, including those of the breast, colon, and reproductive organs. Many hereditary cancer syndromes are characterized by more than one cancer type, so it is important to evaluate the whole family history. The following are some red-flag indicators for further evaluation of high risk syndromes:

- An individual meets revised Bethesda Guidelines. Two of the commonly recognized guidelines are listed here while the guidelines in their entirety can be reviewed in the reference:

  ○ Colorectal cancer before 50 years of age

  ○ Synchronous (multiple-primary cancers present at the same time) or metachronous (second-later cancer), LS-associated tumors (colorectal, endometrial, gastric, ovarian, pancreas, ureter, renal pelvis, biliary tract, brain, and small intestine)

- A family meets Amsterdam criteria (see reference for complete criteria)

  ○ Three relatives with colorectal, endometrial, small bowel, ureter, or renal pelvis cancer in 2 generations, with one diagnosis before 50 years of age

- More than 10 adenomas in one individual

- An individual with multiple GI hamartomas

- An individual from a family with a known hereditary colorectal cancer syndrome

When Would I Want to Refer for a Colonoscopy: Before Genetic Counseling or Testing?

From a statistical standpoint, other pediatric digestive disorders, such as celiac or inflammatory bowel disease are more common. A child with active symptoms that suggest digestive disease (abdominal pain, significant change in bowel habits, rectal bleeding, anemia, or weight loss) should undergo a comprehensive evaluation that may include an endoscopy sooner rather than later.

Bibliography

Clarke AJ, Gaff C. Challenges in the genetic testing of children for familial cancers. *Arch Dis Child.* 2008;93(11):911-914.

National Comprehensive Cancer Network. NCCN clinical practice guidelines in oncology: colorectal cancer screening. v. 2.2011. www.nccn.org

Umar A, Boland CR, Terdiman JP, et al. Revised Bethesda guidelines for hereditary nonpolyposis colorectal cancer (Lynch syndrome) and microsatellite instability. *J Natl Cancer Inst.* 2004;96(4):261-268.

Vasen HF. Clinical diagnosis and management of hereditary colorectal cancer syndromes. *J Clin Oncol.* 2000;18(suppl 1):81S-92S.

QUESTION 48

WHAT IS THE ROLE OF CAPSULE ENDOSCOPY IN PEDIATRICS AND WHAT ARE SOME OTHER NEW OR EMERGING ENDOSCOPIC INNOVATIONS?

Dale Y. Lee, MD and Petar Mamula, MD

Video capsule endoscopy (VCE) is a valuable tool in the evaluation of intestinal pathology. This technology was introduced a decade ago and several devices exist world-wide, 2 of which are available in the United States. Both of these systems utilize radio-frequency technology to remotely transmit images to a capturing device that patients wear for the duration of the study. The design of the capsule varies depending on the target of investigation. For example, VCE can be used to specifically examine the esophagus (in cases of esophageal varices or Barrett's esophagus) or the colon (cancer surveillance). These are more often used in adults; however, a VCE investigation of the small bowel is commonly used in the pediatric population.

VCE involves either ingestion or endoscopic placement of a large, pill-sized camera. The capsule, propelled by intestinal peristalsis, traverses the gastrointestinal (GI) tract and captures images along the way for the duration of the battery life (typically 8 hours). The capsule can be placed endoscopically in patients unable to swallow it, often the case in children aged 7 years and younger due to the capsule's fairly large size (11 mm × 26 to 32 mm). Using proprietary software, the captured images are downloaded and reviewed by a gastroenterologist as a video or enhanced still images. Patients must follow dietary restrictions in order to maximize the chance of complete visualization of the intestinal mucosa. VCE is approved by the Food and Drug Administration for use in the United States in children aged 2 years and older for the evaluation of occult GI bleeding and small bowel Crohn's disease or tumors.

The evaluation of suspected small bowel pathology in pediatric patients is challenging, and commonly requires consultation with a pediatric gastroenterologist. After the initial evaluation including a thorough history, physical examination, laboratory testing, and depending upon symptoms and differential diagnosis, small bowel imaging can be used. Historically, the upper GI series with a small bowel follow-through was commonly used. Lately, this is being replaced by magnetic resonance enterography, targeted small bowel ultrasound, or in select cases, computerized tomographic enterography. These techniques, while often helpful, are limited by not allowing for direct visualization of the intestinal mucosa. Therefore, esophagogastroduodenoscopy (EGD) and colonoscopy are often the next step in evaluation. However, even these techniques are able to evaluate only the very beginning (duodenum) and the very end (terminal ileum) of the small

Table 48-1
Video Capsule Endoscopy: Indications and Findings

Common Indications for Small Bowel VCE	*Other Findings Described in Pediatric Literature*
Occult GI bleeding	Celiac disease
Crohn's disease	Eosinophilic enteropathy
Polyposis syndromes	Lymphangiectasia
	Vascular malformation
	Meckel's diverticulum
	Tumor
	Graft-versus-host disease

bowel, necessitating the need for a diagnostic modality that allows for direct visualization of the entire small bowel.

The most common indications for VCE in pediatrics are occult GI bleeding and inflammatory bowel disease (IBD) (Table 48-1). The evaluation of occult/obscure GI bleed is challenging. If we are presented with a child with anemia and evidence of GI bleeding (either overt or only evidenced by hemoccult positivity), this prompts thorough and expeditious evaluation to determine the source and the severity of bleeding. Patients with serious or life-threatening bleeding are evaluated while hospitalized with a rapid sequence of tests as they are being hemodynamically stabilized. If the source of bleeding cannot be determined through EGD and colonoscopy or imaging studies (eg, tagged red blood cell bleeding scan, Meckel scan, angiography, or computed tomography angiography), a VCE can be a useful tool to determine the source of small bowel bleeding and direct further therapy (Figures 48-1 and 48-2).

IBD is a chronic inflammatory condition causing chronic abdominal pain, diarrhea, hematochezia, and growth failure, among other symptoms. It is currently divided into 2 sub-types: Crohn's disease, which causes discontinuous inflammation of any part of the bowel; and ulcerative colitis (UC), which involves only the colon extending proximally from the rectum. The gold standard for the diagnosis of IBD is histology obtained during an EGD and colonoscopy. In rare instances where such testing is inconclusive, VCE can be used to establish the diagnosis. Additionally, VCE can be used to assess the presence of active small bowel disease in patients with known Crohn's disease, to monitor the degree of mucosal healing in response to Crohn's disease therapy, to evaluate for the presence of small bowel disease in patients with presumed UC (especially prior to planned colectomy), or to further investigate patients when it is not clear if they have Crohn's disease or UC (ie, indeterminate colitis) (Figure 48-3).

Other less common indications for the use of VCE in pediatric patients include evaluation for small bowel polyps in patients with polyposis syndrome or investigation of refractory celiac disease. The utility of VCE in the investigation of chronic abdominal pain, which is one of the most frequent complaints prompting pediatric gastroenterology referral, is very limited.

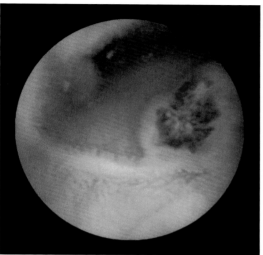

Figure 48-1. Blue rubber bleb nevus syndrome in a 4-year-old patient.

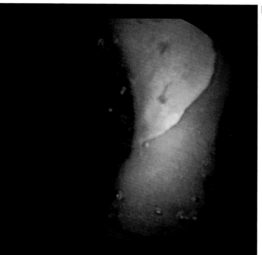

Figure 48-2. Meckel diverticulum and ulcer in a 14-year-old patient.

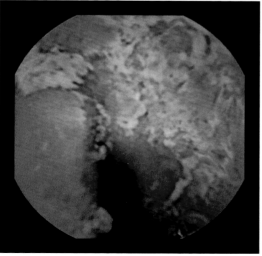

Figure 48-3. Crohn's disease in an 18-year-old patient.

VCE has some notable limitations. The capsule can be retained in the small bowel, requiring endoscopic or surgical removal. Therefore, contraindications to VCE include known small bowel obstruction or stricture, of particular concern in patients with small bowel Crohn's disease. In adults, the rate of capsule retention in Crohn's disease patients is approximately 1%. Pediatric studies are sparse and with only a limited number of subjects. A meta-analysis of pediatric VCE indicated a retention rate of 2.6%. Normal small bowel radiologic imaging is reassuring prior to a VCE study, but it does not exclude the possibility of retention. Another method to prevent capsule retention is the use of a patency capsule. This dissolvable device is similar in size to the VCE, and if passed whole within 36 hours of ingestion, indicates a low risk of retention.

The other limitations of VCE are the inability to obtain tissue for analysis and to perform a therapeutic intervention. There is a great amount of progress being made in the development of new devices that will eventually overcome this limitation. Most of the innovations are at the prototype stage, but some are already available. For example, wireless devices are already used to measure intestinal temperature, pH, pressure, and motility, or capture small bowel images in real-time on a handheld device. Several prototype devices have explored the possibility of mini-robot functionality, including remote maneuverability, collection of specimens, drug delivery via remote puncture of a medication reservoir contained in the capsule, and tissue melding.

Another alternative and nonsurgical method of evaluating the small bowel is double- or single-balloon enteroscopy. This relatively new technique is based on the principle of using balloons and overtubes to navigate an endoscope through the GI tract beyond the third portion of the duodenum, or the terminal ileum. Specifically, the technique employed in this method involves advancement of the instrument by a series of inflating and deflating balloon maneuvers allowing for the anchoring and advancement deep into the small bowel. In select cases, the entire small bowel can be examined this way either using an antegrade, or a combination of the ante- and retrograde approaches. This technique allows for tissue sampling, as well as endoscopic therapeutic interventions to be performed when pathology is detected (eg, polyp removal, bleeding control, or stricture dilation).

Conclusion

VCE is a very useful innovation allowing for direct visualization of the entire small bowel. The indications in pediatric patients mostly involve investigation of small bowel bleeding, IBD, and polyposis syndromes. Further advancements in this field with remotely maneuverable devices and wireless mini-robots will allow us to perform minimally invasive and highly specialized endoscopic interventions within the foreseeable future.

Bibliography

Cohen SA, Klevens AI. Use of capsule endoscopy in diagnosis and management of pediatric patients, based on meta-analysis. *Clin Gastroenterol Hepatol.* 2011;9(6):490-496.

Domagk D, Mensink P, Aktas H, et al. Single- vs. double-balloon enteroscopy in small-bowel diagnostics: a randomized multicenter trial. *Endoscopy.* 2011;43(6):472-476.

El-Matary W. Wireless capsule endoscopy: indications, limitations, and future challenges. *J Pediatr Gastroenterol Nutr.* 2008;46(1):4-12.

Faubion WA, Perrault J. Gastrointestinal bleeding. In: Walker WA, ed. *Pediatric Gastrointestinal Disease.* 3rd ed. Elsevier; New York, New York. 2000:164-178.

Fritscher-Ravens A, Scherbakov P, Bufler P, et al. The feasibility of wireless capsule endoscopy in detecting small intestinal pathology in children under the age of 8 years: a multicentre European study. *Gut.* 2009;58(11):1467-1472.

Sidhu R, Sanders DS, McAlindon ME, Thomson M. Capsule endoscopy and enteroscopy: modern modalities to investigate the small bowel in paediatrics. *Arch Dis Child.* 2008;93(2):154-159.

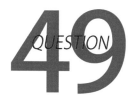

WHY DO SO MANY CHILDREN WITH AUTISM HAVE GASTROINTESTINAL SYMPTOMS AND WHAT ARE THE BEST THERAPIES?

Timothy M. Buie, MD

Autism and autism spectrum disorders (ASD), identified rarely in the past, have had a rising prevalence. The most recent data reported by the Center for Disease Control found autism to be present in 1 in 88 children in the United States. Because the prevalence in boys is almost 5-times higher, 1 in 54 boys and 1 in 252 girls are affected with autism.[1] Autism is characterized by the following:

- Qualitative impairments in social interaction

- Qualitative impairments in communication

- Restrictive, repetitive, and stereotyped patterns of behavior, interests, and activity (DSM-IV)[2]

Many children with ASD also present with sensory processing issues, like hypersensitivity to touch, light, or sound.

Not surprisingly, with the dramatic prevalence of autism noted, there has been great interest in understanding the causes of autism. There is also great interest in exploring the medical issues of children with autism.

Gastrointestinal (GI) problems are commonly described in children with autism; however, many of the problems described are seen in the general pediatric population, as well. A higher frequency of underlying GI pathology in children with autism has not been consistently identified in the published medical literature. In one study, Valicenti-McDermott et al[3] reported that 70% of children with autism had GI problems compared to 42% of children with other neuro-developmental problems, such as cerebral palsy (CP), and 28% of children with typical development. Other studies report a lower frequency of GI problems; Campbell et al[4] reported that 43% of children with autism in a database allowing assessment of medical history had GI problems compared to 4% of unaffected siblings whose data were available.

One other difficulty in assessing this population is that disordered communication is a core component of the diagnosis of autism. Although a caregiver may be able to accurately report stool frequency or consistency, assessing abdominal pain or heartburn is often impossible. Those children with sensory processing abnormalities may have altered pain tolerance, and studies have shown that both hypersensitivity and hyposensitivity to painful stimuli are seen in children with autism. Because of the communication issues, some children may not present with obvious symptoms or complaints. Children with problem behaviors, like aggression or self-injury, may have these issues because of physical pain. These behaviors resolve in some children after treatment for acid reflux, constipation, or other issues. Certainly these behaviors are not limited to GI pain and may occur with otitis, dental pain, and migraine headaches, among others.

The GI issues seen in children with autism are those generally seen in the pediatric population, such as constipation, diarrhea, and gastroesophageal reflux (GER). These conditions are typically evaluated and treated in the same fashion as the general population. The added burden of autism is often the inability to know when treatment is adequate or complete. An unsuccessful trial of antacid for GER may not eliminate heartburn as a possible symptom. More invasive testing is sometimes needed to sort out symptoms. Initial empirical treatments for suspected constipation or reflux often help sufficiently reduce behaviors to support a continued course of treatment. At endoscopy and colonoscopy, some individuals will have inflammation. There does not appear to be a higher frequency of celiac disease (CD) or inflammatory bowel disease (IBD) in this population compared to unaffected children. One speculation is that because of sensory differences, a lesser amount of inflammation could still lead to distress in children with autism.

There has been special interest in the idea that food allergy or intolerance may contribute to autism or behavioral disruption. One mechanism put forward, the opioid peptide theory, suggested that small peptide breakdown products from milk and gluten bind to opioid receptors in the brain, altering behavior and potentially causing autism. This theory has launched attempts to restrict milk and gluten in an effort to improve outcomes. There were open observation studies that suggested a benefit from a gluten-free diet; however, a more recent double-blind study[5] with better design did not show benefit from a casein-free, gluten-free diet. Lactose intolerance has been identified[6] frequently in children with autism undergoing a work-up for GI complaints.

In a consensus report of the medical literature, Buie et al[7] suggested that there is no evidence in the literature to support use of a casein-free, gluten-free diet to treat autism. The article did suggest that there may be children who respond to dietary changes but the mechanism for this is not well understood and needs further study. If families express interest in pursuing dietary changes, involving a nutritionist who has experience with ASD and can provide reasonable goals for diet trials and assuring nutrition is adequate may be helpful.

The question of why so many children with autism have these problems remains unclear. However, recent assessment of the intestinal microbiome has shown differences in the microbiota in children with autism compared with controls. Perhaps these differences contribute to an altered immune or digestive environment.

Another factor that likely contributes to a higher frequency of GI symptoms is the fact that a larger proportion of children with autism present with mitochondrial dysfunction. These children are more likely to suffer motility-related issues, such as GER and constipation. Even in absence of mitochondrial abnormalities, many children with autism have low muscle tone that might also serve as a contributor to bowel dysfunction.

Lastly, there remains a variety of genetic abnormalities seen or suspected in at least a subgroup of children with autism. These genes may have an impact on GI function in some cases. One example is the MET-gene polymorphism described by Campbell et al[8] This abnormality has been identified as an autism promoter and also impacts intestinal healing. Many of the genetic abnormalities seen have yet to be fully characterized in terms of the physical issues that may arise.

Conclusion

GI problems are common in children with autism, and perhaps more so than the general pediatric population. There are unique difficulties in recognizing GI symptoms in children with autism because communication and sensory abnormalities may bring about atypical presentations. There do not seem to be different treatments required for these problems, but perhaps a higher attention for the need of treatment is required for this population. There remain many unanswered questions regarding the cause of GI problems in this condition, and likely there are a number of phenotypes within the diagnosis that make generalization difficult. The challenges in evaluating children with autism can be frustrating, but seeing improvements in these children is profoundly gratifying.

References

1. Centers for Disease Control and Prevention. Prevalence of autism spectrum disorders—autism and developmental disabilities monitoring network. *MMWR*. 2012;61(3):1.
2. Diagnostic and statistical manual of mental disorders (DSM-IV). *Am J Psychiat*. 1994; 866.
3. Valicenti-McDermott M, McVicar K, Rapin I, Wershil BK, Cohen H, Shinnar S. Frequency of gastrointestinal symptoms in children with autistic spectrum disorders and association with family history of autoimmune disease. *J Dev Behav Pediatr*. 2006;27(2 suppl):S128-S136.
4. Campbell DB, Buie TM, Winter H, et al. Distinct genetic risk based on association of MET in families with co-occurring autism and gastrointestinal conditions [published erratum appears in Pediatrics. 2009;123(4):1255]. *Pediatrics*. 2009;123(3):1018-1024.
5. Elder JH, Shankar M, Shuster J, Theriaque D, Burns S, Sherrill L. The gluten-free, casein-free diet in autism: results of a preliminary double blind clinical trial. *J Autism Dev Disord*. 2006;36(3):413-420.
6. Kushak R, Lauwers GY, Winter HS, Buie TM. Intestinal disaccharidase activity in patients with autism: effect of age, gender, and intestinal inflammation. *Autism*. 2011;15(3):285-294.
7. Buie T, Campbell DB, Fuchs GJ 3rd, et al. Evaluation, diagnosis, and treatment of gastrointestinal disorders in individuals with ASDs: a consensus report. *Pediatrics*. 20110;125(suppl 1):S1-S18.
8. Campbell DB, Sutcliffe JS, Ebert PJ, et al. A genetic variant that disrupts MET transcription is associated with autism. *Proc Natl Acad Sci USA*. 2006;103(45):16834-16839.

FINANCIAL DISCLOSURES

Dr. Lindsey Albenberg has no financial or proprietary interest in the materials presented herein.

Dr. Lusine Ambartsumyan has no financial or proprietary interest in the materials presented herein.

Dr. Robert N. Baldassano has no financial or proprietary interest in the materials presented herein.

Dr. William F. Balistreri has no financial or proprietary interest in the materials presented herein.

Dr. Warren P. Bishop has no financial or proprietary interest in the materials presented herein.

Dr. Samra S. Blanchard has no financial or proprietary interest in the materials presented herein.

Dr. Silvana Bonilla has no financial or proprietary interest in the materials presented herein.

Dr. Athos Bousvaros has no financial or proprietary interest in the materials presented herein.

Dr. Timothy M. Buie has no financial or proprietary interest in the materials presented herein.

Dr. Ashley Casserino has no financial or proprietary interest in the materials presented herein.

Dr. Kathy D. Chen has no financial or proprietary interest in the materials presented herein.

Dr. Peter Church has no financial or proprietary interest in the materials presented herein.

Dr. Wallace Crandall has no financial or proprietary interest in the materials presented herein.

Dr. Steven J. Czinn has no financial or proprietary interest in the materials presented herein.

Dr. Marla Dubinsky has no financial or proprietary interest in the materials presented herein.

Dr. Jaime Echartea has no financial or proprietary interest in the materials presented herein.

Dr. Steven H. Erdman receives a research grant from Cancer Prevention Pharmaceuticals.

Dr. Douglas G. Field has no financial or proprietary interest in the materials presented herein.

Dr. Thomas Flass has no financial or proprietary interest in the materials presented herein.

Dr. Alejandro F. Flores has no financial or proprietary interest in the materials presented herein.

Dr. Glenn T. Furuta has no financial or proprietary interest in the materials presented herein.

Dr. Benjamin D. Gold has no financial or proprietary interest in the materials presented herein.

Dr. Tanja Gonska has no financial or proprietary interest in the materials presented herein.

Dr. Nidhi P. Goyal has no financial or proprietary interest in the materials presented herein.

Dr. Anne M. Griffiths is a developer of the PUCAI and receives a share of fees when used in industry-sponsored clinical trials.

Dr. Stefano Guandalini has no financial or proprietary interest in the materials presented herein.

Dr. Sandeep Gupta has no financial or proprietary interest in the materials presented herein.

Dr. Melvin B. Heyman receives grant support relevant to the work from UCB Pharma, Shire Pharma, J & J (Centocor), and NIDDK/NIH.

Dr. Ivor D. Hill has no financial or proprietary interest in the materials presented herein.

Dr. Edward J. Hoffenberg has no financial or proprietary interest in the materials presented herein.

Dr. Jeannie Huang has no financial or proprietary interest in the materials presented herein.

Dr. Sohail Z. Husain has no financial or proprietary interest in the materials presented herein.

Dr. Jeffrey S. Hyams receives research support and a speaker's fee and is on the advisory board for Janssen Ortho Biotech; research support and advisory board for Abbott; and research support and advisory board for Shire.

Dr. Paul E. Hyman has no financial or proprietary interest in the materials presented herein.

Dr. Maureen M. Jonas is a consultant for and receives research support from Roche Pharmaceuticals and receives research support from Schering Plough/Merck.

Dr. Subra Kugathasan has no financial or proprietary interest in the materials presented herein.

Dr. Anayansi Lasso-Pirot has no financial or proprietary interest in the materials presented herein.

Dr. Joel E. Lavine has no financial or proprietary interest in the materials presented herein.

Dr. Dale Y. Lee has no financial or proprietary interest in the materials presented herein.

Dr. Ian Leibowitz has no financial or proprietary interest in the materials presented herein.

Dr. Alan M. Leichtner has no financial or proprietary interest in the materials presented herein.

Dr. Neal S. LeLeiko has no financial or proprietary interest in the materials presented herein.

Dr. Henry Lin has no financial or proprietary interest in the materials presented herein.

Dr. Douglas Lindblad has no financial or proprietary interest in the materials presented herein.

Dr. Debra Lobato has no financial or proprietary interest in the materials presented herein.

Dr. Vera Loening-Baucke has no financial or proprietary interest in the materials presented herein.

Dr. Mark E. Lowe has no financial or proprietary interest in the materials presented herein.

Dr. Laura Mackner has no financial or proprietary interest in the materials presented herein.

Dr. Petar Mamula has no financial or proprietary interest in the materials presented herein.

Dr. Ali A. Mencin has no financial or proprietary interest in the materials presented herein.

Dr. Sonia K. Michail has no financial or proprietary interest in the materials presented herein.

Dr. Jeremy P. Middleton has no financial or proprietary interest in the materials presented herein.

Dr. Douglas Mogul has no financial or proprietary interest in the materials presented herein.

Dr. Michael R. Narkewicz has no financial or proprietary interest in the materials presented herein.

Dr. Catherine D. Newland has no financial or proprietary interest in the materials presented herein.

Dr. Samuel Nurko has no financial or proprietary interest in the materials presented herein.

Dr. Adam Paul has no financial or proprietary interest in the materials presented herein.

Dr. Emily R. Perito has no financial or proprietary interest in the materials presented herein.

Dr. David A. Piccoli has no financial or proprietary interest in the materials presented herein.

Dr. Joel R. Rosh has no financial or proprietary interest in the materials presented herein.

Dr. Audra S. Rouster has no financial or proprietary interest in the materials presented herein.

Dr. Colin Rudolph has no financial or proprietary interest in the materials presented herein.

Dr. Miguel Saps has no financial or proprietary interest in the materials presented herein.

Dr. Shauna Schroeder has no financial or proprietary interest in the materials presented herein.

Dr. Kathleen B. Schwarz receives research funding on HOV from NIDDK, BRSV Roche.

Dr. Jeffrey B. Schwimmer has no financial or proprietary interest in the materials presented herein.

Leigha Senter has no financial or proprietary interest in the materials presented herein.

Dr. Scott H. Sicherer has no financial or proprietary interest in the materials presented herein.

Dr. Natalie Sikka has no financial or proprietary interest in the materials presented herein.

Dr. Edwin F. Simpser has no financial or proprietary interest in the materials presented herein.

Dr. Frank R. Sinatra has no financial or proprietary interest in the materials presented herein.

Dr. Namita Singh has no financial or proprietary interest in the materials presented herein.

Dr. Judith M. Sondheimer has no financial or proprietary interest in the materials presented herein.

Dr. Janis M. Stoll has no financial or proprietary interest in the materials presented herein.

Dr. Alexander Swidsinski has no financial or proprietary interest in the materials presented herein.

Dr. Francisco A. Sylvester has no financial or proprietary interest in the materials presented herein.

Dr. Jonathan E. Teitelbaum is a paid consultant for Danonino, a product by the Dannon Company Incorporated.

Dr. Charles P.B. Vanderpool has no financial or proprietary interest in the materials presented herein.

Dr. Narayanan Venkatasubramani has no financial or proprietary interest in the materials presented herein.

Dr. Dascha C. Weir has no financial or proprietary interest in the materials presented herein.

Dr. Steven L. Werlin has no financial or proprietary interest in the materials presented herein.

Dr. Keith E. Williams has no financial or proprietary interest in the materials presented herein.

Dr. Harland Winter has no financial or proprietary interest in the materials presented herein.

Dr. Nader N. Youssef has no financial or proprietary interest in the materials presented herein.

Dr. Bella Zeisler has no financial or proprietary interest in the materials presented herein.

Index